full of sound

and *fury*

Living with Misophonia

Shaylynn Hayes-Raymond

FULL OF SOUND AND FURY: SUFFERING
WITH MISOPHONIA THIRD EDITION © 2021

imperceptions

Published by Imperceptions Press
Oromocto, New Brunswick, Canada

Cover art and print/eBook design
by East Coast Designs

Originally published under the name Shaylynn Hayes in 2015,
and republished under the author's married name, Shaylynn
Hayes-Raymond.

Ebook ISBN: 978-1-990467-44-8
Print ISBN: 978-1-990467-42-4
Hardcover ISBN: 978-1-990467-43-1

Life's but a walking shadow, a poor player

That struts and frets his hour upon the stage

And then is heard no more.

It is a tale

Told by an idiot, full of sound and fury,

Signifying nothing.

— William Shakespeare

Dedication

Many suffer in silence every day.
This book is for those that need
to know that they're not alone.

Table of Contents

Foreword (2015)

Shaylynn Hayes (now Hayes-Raymond) has written a candid and informative book about misophonia. When I first began to chat with Shaylynn, she reminded me very much of one of my daughters who is the same age. I am very moved by Ms. Hayes' ability to write about this disorder as she shares her own experiences and also takes great care to be objective in presenting both a variety of case studies and different viewpoints about the nature of misophonia.

Ms. Hayes takes misophonia awareness very seriously and has dedicated her time, talent and resources to her book. For Ms. Hayes, misophonia symptoms began at age 16 and as she got older, worsened. For my daughter, they began as far back as I remember.

Over 15 years ago a most amazing 5-year-old child looked at me and asked, "Mommy, can you fix my brain?" She asked me this because she was overly sensitive to noises. These sounds were not necessarily loud, they were not necessarily high-pitched and they were not necessarily noises that other people found aversive or frightening. Yet, for my daughter, these noises were horrifying. They were frightening. They made her angry. My sweet daughter, who was highly social, who loved people, enjoyed being around others and was highly empathic, was stopped dead in her tracks by certain sounds. She became overwhelmed, she had to leave the room, she screamed, she cried, and often I would find her weeping with her hands over her ears in her closet hiding. Could I fix her brain? I couldn't even figure out what sounds were bothering her, never mind why or how to fix the problem.

This began a long journey that has, in essence for me, begun again. When my daughter was 5, after taking her for treatment to a bevy of psychiatrists who misdiagnosed, and mistreated her, I finally figured out what was going on. I was lucky (or perhaps unlucky). I suffer from the same condition. Yet, I don't have it as badly, or at least I didn't when I was younger. Like many others, my symptoms have worsened over time. Yet, having the same symptoms allowed me to figure out what was going on with my daughter.

At the time, around 1996, I was in graduate school studying to be a psychologist, and yet nobody could help my daughter with this "new condition" which was then called Sensory Processing Disorder (SPD). One subtype of the disorder, Sensory Over Responsivity (SOR), describes children who misinterpret sensory information and react to it as though it were aversive. This condition, which includes extreme aversive reactivity to sensory stimuli including sounds, was being studied under the name SPD by Occupational Therapists, not by psychologists and not by psychiatrists. Groundbreaking research by Dr. Lucy Miller and colleagues revealed that auditory and other sensory stimuli are misinterpreted by the brain and cause the sufferer to go into fight/flight. In addition, once the fight/flight response is activated, the part of the nervous system that should put "the brakes on fight/flight" is less efficient. That is, children who are overly sensitive to sensory stimuli react more severely to noise (and other sensory information) and are deficient in calming down.

Fast forward, approximately 18 years later, I have the pleasure of getting to know Ms. Hayes through Facebook groups dedicated to misophonia. Ms. Hayes is a young lady seemingly mature beyond her years, struggling to advocate for and understand this condition. Certain noises and visual triggers make her feel overloaded, out of control, enraged, physically ill, frightened and altogether dysregulated. She, like my daughter, like me and like so many others who have now formed groups on social media, are demanding answers.

Shaylynn is a young lady who has taken advocacy into her own hands by writing a book, a commendable action!

SPD Sensory Over Responsivity? Misophonia or Selective Sound Sensitivity Syndrome? This is not my first "rodeo" with this same or related disorder(s) in which certain sounds (soft ones, repetitive ones, loud ones, ones that go unnoticed by others) are the bane of peoples' existence. I've seen "up close" how the DSM-V rejects SPD and other important disorders for reasons that seem absurd. I've seen firsthand how research does and doesn't get done. I've seen how research is or is not translated into effective therapy.

For me, this is "take two" with what I always called "auditory over- responsivity" but which is now called misophonia. I hope that Ms. Hayes will be an inspiration to others that we must take matters into our own hands. We must not wait for "them to do research" or wait until "they find a cure." There is no "they." We are the "they."

Ms. Hayes, with her high intelligence and ability to reason, fairly and objectively wrote a book that presents differing points of view, while simultaneously revealing real and painful stories of sufferers, including her own.

I hope that people will follow Shaylynn's example and advocate, raise awareness, write books and comment every time they see an article written about misophonia that they don't agree with.

Jennifer Jo Brout – PsyD

Introduction

Welcome to the revised, updated and reworked 2021 edition. The original manuscript of *Full of Sound and Fury* was written in 2015 in an overly ambitious attempt to help spread information on misophonia. In the time since research has grown substantially and understanding and awareness are slowly but surely increasing. Six years later, and I am still advocating for misophonia and promoting education.

With that said, the original edition of *Full of Sound and Fury* is outdated, poorly formatted and essentially a relic of time. I have learned a lot since 2015, and a lot has changed in the world of research and advocacy. The fact that I have to update this book is fantastic because we are no longer out in the wild and research *is* happening! More and more people now know what misophonia is.

The original draft of *Full of Sound and Fury* was full of my fears and anxieties. I worried that research would never pick up, that we would be living without hope for the rest of our lives. I was wrong! This edition supports a new message of education and hope.

What Is Misophonia?

Misophonia (miss-o-phone-e-ah) is known to be a neurological disorder. The term misophonia, literally translating to "hatred of sound," refers to a negative reaction caused by sounds that immediately and involuntarily enrage the sufferer. While the name reflects only sounds, many sufferers are triggered by visuals as well. The condition often leads to isolation, depressed feelings, heightened anxiety, complicated work life and school life and even family and relationship problems. If you are triggered by the mention of trigger sources, please feel free to bypass the following mention of triggers. Most triggers are repetitive actions, and several visual triggers are related to audial triggers. It's important to note that, depending on the person, there can be hundreds of individual triggers. The below are merely examples of common triggers.

Audial Trigger Examples

- Whistling
- Snoring

- Pen-tapping
- Foot-tapping
- Chewing
- Heavy Breathing

Visual Trigger Examples

- Leg shaking
- Swaying
- Bouncing
- Chewing
- Hand movements
- Foot movements
- Pen clicking

An early research study of misophonia interviewed sufferers and, according to the researchers, those with misophonia, "reported feeling offended or violated by these sounds to the point where negative thoughts such as 'I hate this person,' 'Stop it, I can't stand it,' and 'Don't you know what you sound like?' enter their minds" (Edelstein). This reaction is typical for misophonia. Having felt it myself, I can say that no words can describe the intense emotions that happens if you are at the far end of the spectrum.

According to the study "Misophonia: physiological investigations and case descriptions," misophonia is: "a relatively unexplored chronic condition in which a person experiences autonomic arousal (analogous to an involuntary "fight-or-flight" response) to certain innocuous or repetitive sounds such as chewing, pen clicking, and lip smacking. Misophonics report anxiety, panic, and rage when exposed to trigger sounds, compromising their ability to complete everyday tasks and engage in healthy and normal social interaction" (Edelstein).

While this summary leaves out the visual triggers, it is an adequate description of the disorder. Misophonia can be so intense that it interrupts daily life and has caused some sufferers to fall into a deep depression. Sufferers have also expressed reactions from certain fabrics or the sensation of touching certain objects. Other sensory-involved reactions have been documented in cases, and it is clear that these are related. Thus, the name "misophonia" has gotten some flak from both sufferers and members of the medical community. The name "misophonia," meaning hatred of sound, may seem fine to people who relate the disorder to hearing and audial triggers. However, many of the sufferers have problems with visuals as well as tactile problems.

Though some doctors have come up with medical terms and definitions for the disorder, there is no solid evidence or facts that give a solid explanation of what misophonia is.

What we do know is that it should not be assumed that those with misophonia should force exposure to their triggers in order to "get used to them." Any current evidence points to exposure causing the condition to worsen over time. It is important that people with misophonia realize that they should not feel guilty for having the disorder, should know when enough is enough and to leave the situation if they feel that is necessary. Of course, many triggers cannot be avoided entirely, but it is okay to avoid situations that may expose one's self to a high number of them. It is of no use to continue exposing yourself to triggers repeatedly, especially if the reward of the situation or activity is quite low.

Misophonia can feel like a trap. We have been thrown against our will, and without any warrant, in a suffocating prison. Some have suffered their entire lives and, the more fortunate, for a few years. Regardless, the condition is the same. It is important to note that there are several degrees of misophonia.

A lot of the time, a person that has misophonia ends up isolating his or herself from the rest of the world. It can be a heavy burden to be triggered by numerous people and normal activities. This leads to sadness, anxiety and a lowered quality of life. This is especially prominent in individuals who have other disorders – especially mood disorders. Misophonia can cause grief.

Misophonia can do a lot of damage to personal relationships. Misophonia has an impact not only on the sufferer; it also affects the friends, family and romantic partners of the individual. It can cause a lot of arguments and fights and is especially difficult when there is a lack of understanding between persons.

Research

When I wrote the first edition of this book, there were few studies and very few researchers of misophonia. It is delightful to be able to say that this is no longer the case. For a comprehensive review of literature, I suggest you read the academic article from 2018 titled, "Investigating

Misophonia: A Review of the Empirical Literature, Clinical Implications, and a Research Agenda"(https://www.frontiersin.org/articles/10.3389/fnins.2018.00 036/full). While newer studies have come out, this literature review is a great place to start.

There are current notable studies coming out every day, and I am particularly excited by the work by Dr. Sukhbinder Kumar and Mercede Erfanian, "The Motor Basis for Misophonia" (https://www.jneurosci.org/content/41/26/5762). The following significance statement is provided by the study: Conventionally, misophonia, literally "hatred of sounds" has been considered as a disorder of sound emotion processing, in which "simple" eating and chewing sounds produced by others cause negative emotional responses. Our data provide an alternative but complementary perspective on misophonia that emphasizes the action of the trigger-person rather than the sounds which are a byproduct of that action. Sounds, in this new perspective, are only a "medium" via which action of the triggering-person is mirrored onto the listener. This change in perspective has important consequences for devising therapies and treatment methods for misophonia. It suggests that, instead of focusing on sounds, which many existing therapies do, effective therapies should target the brain representation of movement.

As always, up-to-date misophonia research can be found at www.misophonia-research.com as well as www.misophoniaeducation.com which provides presentations with researchers.

My Story

At nineteen years old, I lost my ability to fully take part in the world around me. Unlike common sensory impairments, I did not lose my ability to hear, or smell or see. Instead, I suffer from a condition that amplifies each of these. When I touch, when I look, I am feeling everything around me – and it does not feel pleasant. Imagine you are trapped with the same sound for hours. A slow torture will begin to encapsulate your body. For sufferers of misophonia, a strange yet real condition, this torture is immediate. From the drop of the fork, or the slight pitch of a whistle, we are derailed.

Those that have not heard of misophonia are often surprised by the condition. Some are perplexed by its nature, and have trouble believing that it's more than an annoyance.

For sufferers of misophonia, we are confronted with an immediate fight/flight response to otherwise normal sounds and visuals.

When I first discovered my condition, I went through a lot of emotions. The first was relief that I was not crazy. This was quickly followed by dismay. While I did have a name for the disorder, there was no cure. Soon, my dismay turned to frustration. Information on my disorder, when spread, was often wrong, or even blatantly manipulative. Charlatans were capitalizing off Google, Wikipedia, and the editors at sites as big as WebMD weren't paying attention to scientists. I spent the first year of this disorder wondering what would come of everything – if there was no cure, and no one was paying attention, I didn't know how I was supposed to keep going.

Advocating for an unknown condition is multifaceted. For some, my story has become a beacon, and my efforts are a force to be reckoned with. To many, I have become a symbol of hope. I often feel shame when I sit in my worst moments, void of promise and inspiration. While others look up to me, I spend many moments lost in my own dreariness. The truth is that I am uncomfortable with any idolization for my actions. I am an advocate not for notoriety, but for the ultimate end goal. I am an advocate because I hope for a world that people like me can walk freely upon the streets or have dinner in a restaurant. I am hoping that research, and particularly the wonderful studies that have been championed by Dr. Jennifer Jo Brout, offer more than just a glimmer of hope, but treatment.

While stigma is still a problem for many disorders, I have never had as hard of a time as I do with my disorder that is completely unknown. If I must explain my ADHD, Anxiety or Depression to others, I can point them to research studies—to evidence and proof that these disorders are real. For misophonia, these studies are happening, but at a slow pace, and while there is no treatment, research has picked up in the last 6 years.

I don't mind being an advocate for my disorder. It's invigorating to know that my day-to-day work may have an impact on my own life and that of current and future sufferers. However, that does not mean I am not tired. I am tired of typing, and saying, the same sentence over and over. I am tired of having to justify my disorder whenever I meet a new person. I am tired of explaining why I cannot go to restaurants, or why keys jingling, tapping hands or whistling turn me into a nightmare—crying and all.

When I first discovered what "misophonia" was I had an entirely different story to tell. I was relieved there was a name. I was also scared that I had a disorder that seemed to be under-researched and would be at risk of being stigmatized.

Most people that I have talked to with misophonia have been suffering since they were children. However, I am one of the late bloomers. Regardless of when it came to be, misophonia is an extremely isolating disorder. I was 16 when I showed my first symptoms, but they were not strong. It wasn't until 19 when the full force of misophonia hit me like a freight train. Since then, I have felt its wrath clasp around my throat, taking over several aspects of my life. My first blog post on misophonia was written before I even knew there was a name – before I had anything to go on. I remember writing in frustration, tears not far off, as I wondered why I was so messed up. Why, all of a sudden, I was having so much trouble with sights and sounds. When I first came across misophonia, I described it as ruining my life. I didn't understand why, but these everyday movements and sounds were turning normal situations into a terrible prison.

I attributed my first triggers to an anxiety disorder as well as major depressive disorder. Small movements or rocking back and forth were enough to cause near panic attacks. If a desk was not sitting on the floor properly, I would lose it. If a classmate was making loud, distracting noises, I'd complain to the teacher. It didn't always get me far, but if they didn't help, I'd leave. I wasn't the most attentive student in high school.

On January 27th, 2014, I wrote a post expressing my confusion and rage regarding what I now know as misophonia. Please bear in mind that this was written before I had any idea of what misophonia was. The title was "I don't know what to do." Below, it is recopied in full.

When I first came to university, I didn't remember why I had been so distracted and annoyed in high school. Homework isn't hard, the reading is fine. What I can't deal with is the burden that my anxiety can be in a classroom environment. Half of the time I have a scowl on my face in class and probably come off as a bit of a condescending witch. Whenever people whistle, click their pen, or shake their legs, it's extremely distracting for me and for a reason I cannot explain it sends me into a horrible state. Leg twitching in my peripheral vision has literally brought me to tears. I'm so frustrated that I can't just "get over it". I understand restless leg syndrome is a real thing but so is the anxiety that I suffer every time I enter a classroom. I understand that it would be rude to approach somebody and ask them to please stop torturing me.

Instead, I often stew and try not to get upset but instead I usually just end up irrationally angry. Often times I can actually feel the vibrations on the floor from people shaking behind me, even if they're far away. A couple of weeks ago I started hyperventilating when somebody was whistling. Why? The sharp noise was so unbearable to me. I honestly don't know what I'm supposed to do about this. Breathing exercises, telling myself it's out of my control and "thinking positive" are hopeless. I don't want to constantly glare at my friends like they're the worst thing in the world just because they're shaking their feet. I'm actually sorry it bugs me this much but I can't stop. Sometimes I find myself sitting in my room anxious about going to class just because of my triggers. I just feel alone in this and that I must sound ridiculous to others. Aside from hiding in my room wearing ear plugs and only ever communicating via skype I'm not sure of a fix to this.

My first "real" trigger was whistling. I would go into a rage and nearly cry whenever faced with it. Some people would whistle on purpose, because they did not understand the severity of my reaction. I remember being upset for hours after this would happen, and that confused me a lot. Then, one day, my mother's foot-shaking really started to bother me. Soon after, the sound of singing and country music really sent me over the edge. This caused a lot of fights and confusion. Why was I so intolerant? It made no sense to me.

While there are many triggers that seem to pop up in numerous people, not everybody has the same triggers. We're not all the same, so that makes it even harder to raise awareness. However, regardless of what a person is triggered by, we're still triggered, and it can be very disorienting.

It's hard for me not to think of Shakespeare's quote, "full of sound and fury signifying nothing." This quote perfectly expresses the disorder, and that's why it's been incorporated into the title. There's no logical reason to freak out—we can feel crazy, guilty and downright ridiculous. It's full of fury. The simple clicking of a pen can feel like we're trapped in a cavern with a jackhammer.

Melodrama aside, I believe that a good life is possible with misophonia and even more possible with the right coping skills. I am no longer afraid of misophonia, and I truly believe that there is a lot of hope to be had!

Full of Sound and Fury

Interviews With Sufferers

People whose lives are affected by misophonia filled out the following interviews graciously. All of the answers are unaltered, with the exception of spelling or grammar, and are 100% honest. The opinions within these interviews are that of the interviewees. The question form was the same for each individual. The following interviews are not presented in any given order. I am so thankful to the people who chose to share their experiences with misophonia in this book.

Full of Sound and Fury

Interview 1: Adam Johnson

At what age did you start to have triggers for misophonia?

I have a clear memory at about 7 years old with a single trigger.

What are your top 5 triggers?

- Chewing of any kind (both auditory and visual)
- Breathing
- Fingers on keyboards
- Sipping / slurping (assuming this is different than chewing, and auditory only)
- Bright lights (reflections, point sources, etc.)

What is worse, visual triggers or audial triggers?

Audial is much more severe. Bright lights are right behind and are a migraine trigger as well.

When did you learn that there was a name for your condition and other sufferers?

About 2 years ago I found the term Selective Sound Sensitivity Syndrome online. This led me to misophonia.

How did it feel to learn that there were other people like you?

It made me feel better for sure. This sensitivity can make me hard to live and work with sometimes, so it made me feel less... crazy?

How do you cope with this disorder?

When eating with family and friends, I make sure to have music playing to minimize the eating sounds. Restaurants are chosen for the same reason. I wear headphones a lot. A whole lot. This drowns out keyboards in offices, people on airplanes, etc. For the light sensitivity part, I wear sunglasses a lot, keep offices and living spaces free of bright lights, and arrange computer screens to not reflect.

Are your family and friends supportive?

No. It's not an easy thing to grasp, and I just seem like I'm being annoyed.

Are you afraid to confront a person when they are triggering you?

Unfortunately, I confront often. I ask people (and many times strangers) to stop slurping coffee, to chew with their mouths closed, to spit out their gum, etc.

If a person does not respect your condition, how do you react?

I have to leave before I take their coffee, food, gum away.

Do you have other disorders that worsen your misophonia?

When I'm feeling "migraine-prone," which I consider unusually light-sensitive and not far from triggering a migraine, my sensitivity to all things intensifies.

Do you think the name suits the disorder? Why? Why not?

Yes. Sound is often my enemy and I therefore hate it. This is unfortunate for the people creating the sounds...

What do you think could be done to raise awareness?

Perhaps some legitimate interviews on mainstream media with legitimate medical professionals.

Explain the reaction when faced with a trigger:

I first try to just ignore it, to focus on something else. If it continues and I start to feel either pain and/or anger, I see if it's something I can fix delicately, or if I need to take myself out of the situation. If I'm 'stuck' in the environment and glaring at someone isn't working and I can't discretely plug my ears, a last resort is to try to explain that sounds are hurting me. Either way, the longer the sound goes on, the more I go from mildly annoyed and patient, to pained, to downright angry and irrational.

Interview 2: Simone Zoffmann Johansen

At what age did you start to have triggers for misophonia?

I first really noticed when I was 14 years old, which is 4 years ago.

What are your top 5 triggers?

It's hard for me to categorize the triggers in numbers, but my worst triggers are:

- People chewing – basically everything is annoying me about that
- People making a noise with candy bags, chips bags, etc.
- People using their mouse pad on their computers or using their keyboard. People playing with a pen, clicking it etc.
- People making a noise with their fingers on a table rhythmically

What is worse, visual triggers or audial triggers?

Audial triggers are for sure the worst kinds of triggers, but the hard thing is that, when you start getting anxiety of audial triggers, visual triggers can be just as horrible as audial triggers because inside your head you can hear the audial triggers when you get visually triggered.

When did you learn that there was a name for your condition and other sufferers?

About a half year ago, by a coincidence, I found a Danish name for the condition which is called "to be particularly sensitive." It was at first a huge relief. I read a whole lot about it and it was fantastic to find out that I wasn't the only one who was triggered by something. Someday, again by a coincidence, one of my classmates (who I have yelled at many times, because he has triggered me with his noises) came and showed me a so-called meme from Facebook which said, "getting angry at people when hear them breathing or eating is called 'misophonia', which is an actual brain disorder." Then I researched a lot about misophonia and found out that this was the word which described everything that I felt inside.

How did it feel to learn that there were other people like you?

It was a huge relief. Day in and day out for at least 4 years I have been called a lot of things for being so rude, angry, parochial and hysterical. Suddenly there was an explanation which I, more than anyone else, had been searching for because you start asking a lot of questions about if it is your own fault, and if you are strange, etc.

How do you cope with this disorder?

It is very hard on a daily basis to be in a normal school and listen to the teacher, while you are trying to ignore all the triggers. Also, the family life is very hard to struggle with because if you think getting triggered on a normal basis is hard, you should try being triggered by someone you care about.

Some days are good and some days are bad. That is pretty much how I cope with it. Sometimes you just need a break from the life and people. And then you have to take one day at a time and really be patient with yourself and try to count to ten at least 30 times a day.

Are your family and friends supportive?

It's only the closest part of my family who know about misophoni, and they are being very supportive. I'm not sure how I feel about telling others because I think that it is seen as a weakness and I'm afraid how people would react and think.

Are you afraid to confront a person when they are triggering you?

I'm very afraid to confront people who are triggering me because I don't want them to look at me and think that I am annoying, so I don't confront people.

If a person does not respect your condition, how do you react?

I get upset and sad because then they know that they are hurting me and suddenly it's on purpose.

Do you have other disorders that worsen your misophonia?

No.

Do you think the name suits the disorder? Why? Why not?

I think that it's a fine name. Actually, I'm just glad that there is a name for it that I know and that other people in the same situation know.

What do you think could be done to raise awareness?

I really don't know. If I knew I would probably already be doing it, but at this moment where I'm too scared to even tell my family, how could I tell the world?

Explain the reaction when faced with a trigger:

My stomach hurts. My concentration is 110% focused on the trigger noise, and I cannot get it away from there. I'm starting to feel the tears in my eyes and just try to hold them back. I get the feeling of sadness, anger and I want to hit someone (myself, basically). There comes a time where I no longer can stay in the situation and in the room and then I have to leave. If I don't leave, I can just sit and wait for the noise to go away, trying to not let my tears get through.

Full of Sound and Fury

Interview 3: Victoria

At what age did you start to have triggers for misophonia?

My first serious trigger was when I was about 8 when I was staying at my aunt's house, she claimed she didn't know she was chewing in my ear though it was impossible for her not to notice the angle she was sitting at. Before this, it was very mild – I did notice all my triggers but they were almost non-existent until my aunt did this. As a result, I used to get grounded and banned from things because I told people to shut up when they were eating.

What are your top 5 triggers?

- Any form of food in someone's mouth – even my own
- Gulping – food and liquids
- Hearing mucus in someone's nose – especially when I'm eating
- Whistling
- Biting nails

What is worse, visual triggers or audial triggers?

All of the above plus people sliding their fingers on guitar strings, also foot-tapping – worst is people shaking their feet so violently one might think their foot might fall off.

When did you learn that there was a name for your condition and other sufferers?

In February 2015 through Facebook.

How did it feel to learn that there were other people like you?

I felt relieved that I wasn't going crazy, I was told I had to go and get medical help because I was supposed to have something mentally wrong with me like some sort of lunatic because it was causing problems at home, but as soon as I found out about this in February, I posted it all over Facebook to prove to certain people who won't be named that I am not the psychopath they were making me out to be.

I still can't describe how happy I am now that I can put a name to this.

How do you cope with this disorder?

I often have to remove myself from the situation before I get the compulsive urge to punch someone. I also have to excuse myself from other people's houses as soon as possible so I don't do or say something that I will end up regretting.

Are your family and friends supportive?

No, they all think I'm still crazy and that I am using this to cause arguments.

Are you afraid to confront a person when they are triggering you?

I've had certain people tell me that I would get my face slapped if I did.

If a person does not respect your condition, how do you react?

Unfortunately, I have to bite my tongue in most situations, other people I will excuse myself and politely explain why I feel uncomfortable, it's their choice how they want to take that.

Do you have other disorders that worsen your misophonia?

Severe depression.

Do you think the name suits the disorder? Why? Why not?

Well, it does translate to hatred of noise, so, yeah, I suppose it does.

What do you think could be done to raise awareness?

I think there should be more charities and events and stuff to not only raise awareness but to also help provide the right support for those who don't have it at home, a good example would be a weekly meeting in a local library or have a charity café of sorts.

Explain the reaction when faced with a trigger:

The reaction I have is to punch someone so hard they think twice before setting my trigger off again, the worse the trigger is the worse my fight and flight is. Other than telling people to shut up as a child I have only ever lashed out once (verbally thankfully) asking the person to spit their gum out as they were chewing in my ear (not my aunt this time), I was in the middle of an exam at the time, so I had to really bite my tongue hard to not get up and lamp them one.

Interview 4: Jami Blackwell

At what age did you start to have triggers for misophonia?

9

What are your top 5 triggers?

Gum cracking, sniffing, smacking, tapping, whistling and throbbing bass (sorry, there's 6).

What is worse, visual triggers or audial triggers?

Audial.

When did you learn that there was a name for your condition and other sufferers?

About two and a half years ago.

How did it feel to learn that there were other people like you?

I felt relief and validation.

How do you cope with this disorder?

Mostly by avoidance or covering it with a louder noise like my big fan or turn up the TV.

Are your family and friends supportive?

My husband and kids are. Growing up, I was just called crazy.

Are you afraid to confront a person when they are triggering you?

It depends on the trigger.

If a person does not respect your condition, how do you react?

I get highly irritated, but I try not to let it show and escape the situation as quickly as I can.

Do you have other disorders that worsen your misophonia?

No.

Do you think the name suits the disorder? Why? Why not?

Yes, because it is a pretty much straightforward definition.

What do you think could be done to raise awareness?

I am not sure. Maybe some documentaries or quick ads about it on TV...

Explain the reaction when faced with a trigger:

I pretty much go to instant rage ... especially if it is a rudeness thing. It isn't necessary for one to play his bass so loudly that the siding on my house vibrates. It isn't necessary for one to let his child play the drums on the chairs at church in the middle of church services. Stuff like that is just plain rude and causes instant rage. I leave the situation. It is still bad, but not quite so bad, if the trigger isn't such an outright rudeness thing.

Full of Sound and Fury

Interview 5: Senta K Baker

At what age did you start to have triggers for misophonia?

15

What are your top 5 triggers?

Gum chewing, lip smacking, sniffling, eating with mouth open, and chomping ice.

What is worse, visual triggers or audial triggers?

Both have the same effect on me.

When did you learn that there was a name for your condition and other sufferers?

Two years ago while watching 60 minutes TV Show.

How did it feel to learn that there were other people like you?

Started searching the Internet when I learned there was a name and found the Facebook group.

How do you cope with this disorder?

I flee, I remove myself and have recently begun using headphones.

Are your family and friends supportive?

I hid this from all of my friends until a couple of years ago. I told my boss and sometimes I feel like that was a mistake. My two girls both suffer from it but on different levels and my granddaughter (3) also suffers from it but my daughter is in denial.

Are you afraid to confront a person when they are triggering you?

I so want to lash out but I just remove myself.

If a person does not respect your condition, how do you react?

My second husband was horrible, knew chomping ice set me over the edge and he was mean about it, so I would remove myself.

Do you have other disorders that worsen your misophonia?

Not that I'm aware of.

Do you think the name suits the disorder? Why? Why not?

I haven't really thought about it, either way, I'm just happy there is a name for it.

What do you think could be done to raise awareness?

PSA, news articles that Joe Public would see, not just scholarly journals.

Explain the reaction when faced with a trigger noise:

This past weekend I was shopping in a local drug store and there was a woman who was chewing her gum like there was no tomorrow, could almost see her molars. So, I kept dodging her throughout the entire store even though I was ready to check out I had to make sure I wasn't in earshot or a visual. Waited until she checked out and then made my way, but then the gal at the counter was eating chips, I just about died. Hoping to get a survey later from the store so I could complain about employees eating while waiting on customers.

Full of Sound and Fury

Interview 6: Alkisti Karakoli

At what age did you start to have triggers for misophonia?

Around puberty.

What are your top 5 triggers?

People chewing with their mouth open. Lip smacking. Teeth sucking. Gulping while drinking. Pigeons. High pitched women's voices with long vowels and whistling 's' letters.

What is worse, visual triggers or audial triggers?

Audial.

When did you learn that there was a name for your condition and other sufferers?

A few years ago (2 or 3) I read an article about it on the Internet.

How did it feel to learn that there were other people like you?

It was a huge relief. I always thought I was just being weird about it and couldn't really understand why I was reacting so badly. That is, when the trigger sound stopped.

How do you cope with this disorder?

I am honest to the ones triggering me when I think they will understand. Otherwise, I try to leave the area or cover my ears. I also avoid going to places like the cinema.

I haven't found a solution about the pigeon problem.

Are your family and friends supportive?

Some of them are and some of them aren't. There are also those that seem to understand me when I explain my situation but still trigger me as they don't realize the sounds they produce.

Are you afraid to confront a person when they are triggering you?

When the trigger is 'on' I can't say I am able to have a conversation about it. I am just mad. I avoid confrontation since I know I will regret my rage afterwards. Sometimes, I can't hold it, though.

If a person does not respect your condition, how do you react?

It depends. If it's a random person I just go away or avoid people like that in general.

If it's someone close to me (like my father – it's not that he does not respect my condition, he falls in the category of people that do not realize the sounds they make) I try to find ways to be around him. Like having the TV on while we eat together, or leave the area when he has a snack etc.

Do you have other disorders that worsen your misophonia?

No, I don't think I do.

Do you think the name suits the disorder? Why? Why not?

Not really. Since it's of Greek origin, the definition of the combined words is "hatred of voice" and that is not accurate for sounds other than voices.

What do you think could be done to raise awareness?

I think we need a medical proof that something we can't help is wrong with us. Otherwise, when I think about it, I understand it's really difficult for people not experiencing this to understand we are not some kind of angered freaks.

Explain the reaction when faced with a trigger:

When the trigger starts, I feel my brain is searching the area to hear the sound again. Is it there? Is it not there? Do I hear something? When it does, it locks on that direction. Then it's almost all I can hear. The expression that comes to my mind about this is "target fixation" (I got that from motorcycle riding, but it fits). After that I split in two. One part of me is looking for ways to avoid the sound and the other wants to keep hearing it ... it's like a part of me wants to get annoyed ... and angry ... and furious. I grit my teeth and make fists with my hands. Sometimes I bang the desk in front of me (if there is a desk) before realizing I'm doing it. I want to attack the source and scream. I glance angrily, I feel ... possessed. My breathing changes and I really hate the source.

When the source is someone I love, I feel so very sorry afterwards. The guilt makes me sad. Makes me cry. Who am I? What is that?

I think I've made some progress though. After experiencing this rage and guilt so many times in my life, I know what's coming when the trigger starts, so I usually choose the 'flight' solution. When I stay and try to endure it ... sometimes the 'magnitude' of an incident can still surprise me. So, nope, it's not really me. But it's something I have.

Full of Sound and Fury

Interview 7: Ella Orr

At what age did you start to have triggers for misophonia?

I think I was about 7 or 8. I was cuddling up against my mum on the sofa and she started to eat a banana sandwich. I remember feeling really bothered by the sound.

What are your top 5 triggers?

- Wet mouth noises of all kinds, even the merest sound when someone parts their lips
- Chewing, visual and auditory – worst when open-mouthed, but still pretty bad when closed-mouthed
- Crunching
- Throat-clearing
- Audible breathing through nose (especially when there is a whistling sound)

What is worse, visual triggers or audial triggers?

Auditory triggers.

When did you learn that there was a name for your condition and other sufferers?

In my late 20s. I was curled up in bed, crying my eyes out about having to go for dinner with some relatives who were terrible about eating with their mouths open. My husband was so concerned he Googled it and came and told me about what he found.

How did it feel to learn that there were other people like you?

It was a massive relief, like a huge burden lifted from my shoulders. Beforehand I thought I was out of order for getting so annoyed. I'd beat myself up for being unreasonable and too easily irritated. I thought I was being stupid and that I was just an unpleasant person, or maybe slightly mad. When I read about the disorder online, I started crying again – seeing people articulating the exact same things that went on in my head, with the same triggers and reactions, reassured me that it wasn't just me, and that there was actually a reason for my behavior.

How do you cope with this disorder?

I wear earplugs at night. I listen to loud music using earphones whenever I'm on public transport. At work, if someone near me starts eating, I try and close off the nearest ear by making it look like I'm leaning on my hand, or I'll nip out to the toilets or to the kitchen. Basically, I cope by blocking out or running away whenever it's possible.

Are your family and friends supportive?

My husband is incredibly supportive. I have also told a couple of my closest, most open-minded friends, and my mum. They are all good about it. Other than that, I don't tell people. I tried for a while, but I found that after spending so much of my life bottling up the anger and keeping the suffering inside, I'm not good at talking about it.

Are you afraid to confront a person when they are triggering you?

Yes. I very rarely do this. I still see it as being my problem rather than theirs. I fear coming across as whiny, irritable. I can't fully explain to them how it makes me feel.

If a person does not respect your condition, how do you react?

Mostly I consider it my fault for not explaining it properly. Sometimes, after I have tried, the person will seem sympathetic and interested and understanding – but their eating habits don't change. I can't blame them for forgetting.

Do you have other disorders that worsen your misophonia?

I don't think so.

Do you think the name suits the disorder? Why? Why not?

As a literal description, it's fine. I'm wary about making it come across as a phobia though.

What do you think could be done to raise awareness?

I really don't know. If there was some comparison we could make - non-sufferers can't empathize if they have no way of relating. My husband describes it like being able to hear pain. It's difficult to get people to care about something so utterly unfathomable. Explain the reaction when faced with a trigger:

The second I hear the tiniest trigger sounds, it's as if my entire concentration involuntarily latches on and focuses in on it. I always try to look outwardly normal, but a close observer might see that I'm gritting my teeth, pursing my lips, twitching my foot, scratching my arm ... these are all signs that internally, I'm absolutely losing it. If I can't escape it, for example at a dinner table, my heart rate increases, my stomach drops, my head spins. It's an intense level of agitation and discomfort. Most of all, it's an overwhelming feeling of anger, of rage. If I look up and see a person eating their food with their mouth open, for that moment right there, I passionately hate them. In my head, I'll be screaming. I often think I would genuinely prefer physical pain. I rage against the person causing the trigger to a ridiculous degree. But – as soon as I'm free of the situation and the trigger is gone – all of those feelings disappear with it and are replaced with crippling shame. I'll feel ridiculous, mean, crazy. I'll think about my actions in trying to deal with it, like covering my ears, beating up my computer mouse to drown it out, sitting as far as humanly possible away from everyone else at the table – and they'll feel stupidly obvious. Even though at the time I couldn't have cared less about my actions looking weird to other people. When it's happening, I want the offender to notice me, to know I despise them, so they will just stop. Once the situation is over, I immediately feel terrible and full of regret and shame. It's like being temporarily mad.

Interview 8: Lauren Fletcher

At what age did you start to have triggers for misophonia?

The earliest I remember is around age 10.

What are your top 5 triggers?

The sound of someone chewing, especially crunchy foods; gum chewing or popping; smacking or slurping; repetitive coughing, nasal sounds or open-mouth breathing; repetitive clicking or tapping sounds.

What is worse, visual triggers or audial triggers?

Audial.

When did you learn that there was a name for your condition and other sufferers?

About a year ago. Until then, I thought there was something profoundly wrong with just me.

How did it feel to learn that there were other people like you?

I felt relieved. I stumbled across articles and Kelly Ripa's ABC interview via Pinterest and started crying at my work desk. My therapist had been suggesting that perhaps the sound sensitivity was rooted in my eating disorder or PTSD; she had never heard of misophonia until after I told her about the articles I'd read.

How do you cope with this disorder?

I internalize a lot. I wear earplugs when I'm in the car with my husband so I don't hear him breathing or making noises. I avoid places where I know there will be triggers. I give myself time limits in meetings so I know that I don't have to endure pen-clicking or mint-chewing for an extended amount of time. I keep the door closed to my office, and keep the fan on and earbuds in so I don't hear people walking by, eating or popping their gum. I wear ear plugs to the movie theatre, during dinner with my family, on planes or really any place where someone could be eating or making trigger sounds.

Are your family and friends supportive?

Somewhat. Though I've told my parents and husband about the disorder, they seem relatively oblivious to the sounds they make that bother me. My best friend does a good job of being cognizant regarding my triggers.

Are you afraid to confront a person when they are trigger ng you?

Yes.

If a person does not respect your condition, how do you react?

I internalize and stay away from them.

Do you have other disorders that worsen your misophonia?

I have Social Anxiety disorder and Obsessive-compulsive Personality disorder. I'm not sure if they worsen the misophonia, or vice versa, or if one is the result of the other. I would love to know.

Do you think the name suits the disorder? Why? Why not?

I understand the scientific significance of the name, but I'm not sure the general public would hear or read it and know that it involves hearing and/or anger. Sometimes I think the word "audio" should be included somewhere since people usually associate that with hearing more so than the "-phonia" suffix.

What do you think could be done to raise awareness?

There needs to be active discussion in the medical/psychological community about adding this disorder to the DSM. There need to be articles in medical and health journals. More people with the disorder need to start speaking out about what they live with. Audiologists and psychotherapists need to start establishing relationships with each other to co-treat their patients.

Explain the reaction when faced with a trigger:

I get tunnel vision – I can't focus on anything else but that noise. Even when it's not actively happening, I am bracing myself for when it will which increases my anxiety. When I hear the noise, the reaction in my body is the same as if I've been hit or physically injured; I tense up and feel a burning sensation in my stomach. I have the overwhelming need to run away, but the rational part of me makes me stay where I am because I know it's just a noise. I find myself giving dirty looks or exasperated stares towards the person making the noise. I am snippy with my words and my tone. I clinch my fists and try not to make eye contact with the trigger person. I think about hitting them or yelling at them to stop making the sound.

Full of Sound and Fury

Interview 9: Ashley

At what age did you start to have triggers for Misophonia?

> 6-7 years old.

What are your top 5 triggers?

> Gum popping, food smacking/crunching, constant throat clearing, coughing, open-mouth eating.

What is worse, visual triggers or audial triggers?

> Audial.

When did you learn that there was a name for your condition and other sufferers?

> 2012, approximately.

How did it feel to learn that there were other people like you?

> It was a huge relief. It made me feel hopeful that I could overcome this disorder.

How do you cope with this disorder?

I have a strong "flight" response. I leave if I can. If not, I just try my best to go to my "happy place" and tell myself that it will be over eventually.

Are your family and friends supportive?

My fiancé is super supportive. He really tries to eat quietly and to make noise when other people aren't. My parents are trying to understand, but they will slip sometimes and get annoyed when I have to leave during a meal.

Are you afraid to confront a person when they are triggering you?

Yes, I have had some negative experiences when trying to be honest about the condition. I've heard responses like 'how dare you judge how I eat?' or 'you're making me feel self-conscious.'

If a person does not respect your condition, how do you react?

I refuse to be around them if I don't need to while eating.

Do you have other disorders that worsen your misophonia?

I suffer from anxiety, but I truly feel like the misophonia is the same no matter how I am feeling.

Do you think the name suits the disorder? Why? Why not?

I think it's perfect. I absolutely hate some sounds.

What do you think could be done to raise awareness?

More doctors need to specialize in the disease. People won't take it seriously unless they feel like it's a real condition.

Explain the reaction when faced with a trigger:

At first, I'm in shock. I'm shocked that a person cannot control their actions/noises and I feel personally offended. I will usually stare at the person, if I can without them noticing. Then I'm disgusted and I will get angry. Some people can tell that I'm angry because I will become quiet and I will start to fidget. Then the panic (or flight) response happens. If I can, I will leave immediately. Then I usually feel guilty.

Full of Sound and Fury

Interview 10: Vera

At what age did you start to have triggers for misophonia?

I am not 100% sure but it was definitely between the ages of 7-10.

What are your top 5 triggers?

My triggers: When my mother says the letter S, and then visual with her is pointing or talking with hands-type thing. My brother, it's his coughing, sniffling (throat noises) and visual it's when he shuffles his feet or wiggles his toes (leg movements). Just recently my BF started to trigger me and for him it's his throat noises also ... but, nothing else just yet.

What is worse, visual triggers or audial triggers?

They are both equally as annoying. For me it's been audial. I don't have many visual triggers but if I did, I would personally get more bothered by the visuals. Noises there are headphones or sound blockers but for visuals you literally just have to look away or leave the room.

When did you learn that there was a name for your condition and other sufferers?

Probably a year or two ago ... I think my dad might have mentioned it before. But I hadn't really looked into it until this year. There's a lot more awareness and people coming out just these past 2 years alone.

How did it feel to learn that there were other people like you?

Umm ... I felt like finally there are people I can talk to that will just get it. I have super supportive friends and family, but it feels great to know people just get it. It's also very hopeful and helpful learning people's experiences and coping mechanism.

How do you cope with this disorder?

Counting my blessings, my family and friends are willing to understand and compromise. My misophonia is only with certain people also, which has made the case less severe. HEADPHONES and SOOTHING SOUNDS or just MUSIC are key to life with misophonia. I also try and maintain a positive attitude, good eating habits, good exercise habits, etc. I don't know if it helps but what I do know is when I am stressed, my triggers are 10x.

Are your family and friends supportive?

Yes, they try the best they can.

Are you afraid to confront a person when they are trigger ng you?

No, that's the last thing I am afraid of. As terrible as this sounds, if I didn't have control over my stress and anxiety, I'd be smacking everyone. But I politely tell them to stop or I plug myself into headphones.

If a person does not respect your condition, how do you react?

I've never encountered that just yet, my triggers aren't with random strangers. But I would just find them to be ignorant.

Do you have other disorders that worsen your misophonia?

I don't think so ... stress is what really gets me. If I have a nice relaxing day my triggers are pretty under control but if it's been stressful, it's like a crapshoot.

Do you think the name suits the disorder? Why? Why not?

Yeah ... I think so.

What do you think could be done to raise awareness?

I think people should be going to offices, schools etc. where people have to work and deal with this condition in everyday life. It educates the person suffering and the people around them.

Explain the reaction when faced with a trigger:

I feel anger, sadness and stress. But I constantly have to remind myself it's not them nor me it's the misophonia monster.

Interview 11: Sharon Mousel

At what age did you start to have triggers for misophonia?

10.

What are your top 5 triggers?

- "S" sounds
- Foot-tapping
- Chewing/gulping/smacking
- Slurping
- Fork hitting teeth

What is worse, visual triggers or audial triggers?

Audial.

When did you learn that there was a name for your condition and other sufferers?

Age 15.

How did it feel to learn that there were other people like you?

It felt amazing. It kind of made misophonia valid to me.

How do you cope with this disorder?

I use earplugs and headphones. I took magnesium for a little bit, but it didn't work out for me.

Are your family and friends supportive?

Yes.

Are you afraid to confront a person when they are triggering you?

No. I'm not afraid, but I don't confront people if they are triggering me, I just leave if I can. The reason why is because I know asking someone, "Please, stop breathing" or "Please, stop eating like a pig," will seem very irrational to someone. Unless I'm wearing my bracelet that says "Misophonia Awareness," I'd show it to them and just bring up a conversation about it, and tell them I have it.

If a person does not respect your condition, how do you react?

Fortunately, I haven't encountered someone I don't know who disrespected my condition. Back in the day though, my dad and my aunt were not supportive of my condition, and since I couldn't tell them what I had—

because I didn't know—they thought I was being bratty and kept triggering me.

Do you have other disorders that worsen your misophonia?

Not that I know of.

Do you think the name suits the disorder? Why? Why not?

While "misophonia" is the more popular name (and I use it a lot), I do prefer "Selective Sound Sensitivity Syndrome" if I was to introduce it to someone I've never met before. It sounds more professional, I think. I would also mention the term "misophonia" and that it is more popularly known as that.

What do you think could be done to raise awareness?

I put on a T-shirt campaign and many of my family members bought a shirt. I hope it spreads awareness. I think bracelets are a more efficient way to spread awareness, however. I also did a research report on it for a class, so my teacher became aware of it. I also tell my teachers ahead of time that I may need to wear headphones during class, and I would explain I have misophonia.

Explain the reaction when faced with a trigger:

At first, it's anxiety, but that's only if I know someone is going to, say, slurp a cup of coffee in front of me. Next, it's anger. Extreme anger. And I sometimes hit something if it's really bad. When it's all said and done, I feel tired and slightly moody.

Interview 12: Victoria MacNeil-LeBlanc

At what age did you start to have triggers for misophonia?

Around age 10 or so, but I do have one memory of reacting very negatively to my father whistling when I was 6 or 7 years old.

What are your top 5 triggers?

Gum and general open-mouthed chewing, nail biting, loud breathing, finger and foot tapping and nail picking.

What is worse, visual triggers or audial triggers?

Audial triggers, but I am affected by visual triggers as well.

When did you learn that there was a name for your condition and other sufferers?

I read about it in a "weird personality quirks that are actually medical conditions" article online (on Cracked) when I was 15 years old, in May 2013.

How did it feel to learn that there were other people like you?

It felt great to learn that I'm not a rude, controlling person, and I'm not the only one. My parents thought that I was a controlling brat, it was nice to learn that my behavior had an explanation and was not inappropriate.

How do you cope with this disorder?

Asking my parents/friends to stop triggering me, always having earplugs/headphones with me, avoiding specific people/events that trigger me.

Are your family and friends supportive?

Mostly. My dad can get pretty angry sometimes when I ask him to stop triggering me, especially when it's a visual trigger, but I know that, ultimately, he wants me to be happy and healthy. My mom is supportive but gets mad if I "sound angry" when I ask her to stop triggering me. Otherwise, they're nice and supportive, probably around 97% of the time. My best friend is the only other person who knows, and she's supportive.

Are you afraid to confront a person when they are triggering you?

Yes, I've never confronted anyone except for my parents and best friend, and probably never would. I'm very shy.

If a person does not respect your condition, how do you react?

With anger internally, but externally I try to remain calm and respond in a sophisticated, intelligent way in an attempt to almost shame them for their ignorance and inability to respect invisible diseases/disorders.

Do you have other disorders that worsen your misophonia?

No. I have OCD and a few other issues but I don't believe that any of them make my misophonia any worse.

Do you think the name suits the disorder? Why? Why not?

Yes, I do. I only wish that misophonia didn't literally mean hatred of sounds, because saying I have the hatred of sounds when trying to explain my visual triggers is very awkward and nearly impossible to explain.

What do you think could be done to raise awareness?

I'd like to see misophonia discussed more often on the radio/TV, but it must be done with respect. I've heard a local radio station (104.5 Chum FM) make fun of misophonia, purposely triggering a woman by making loud chewing/ slurping noises into the microphone while she tried to explain it to the DJ. It was disgusting and hurtful, and probably set the misophonia movement back a few years by making thousands of listeners think that it's just a joke. So, if misophonia could be addressed with respect by the media that would be great. If I ever get rich, I'm going to put out commercials and advertisements about misophonia, seriously.

Explain the reaction when faced with a trigger:

I feel immediate disgust and anger ... I need it to stop, somehow. If it's a parent or friend, I ask them to stop. I try to be respectful and polite but it often comes out sounding rude because I'm angry. A lot of misophonia sufferers have issues with controlling their anger when they're being subjected to a trigger, but few non-sufferers understand this and take offense. If it's someone I can't talk to, I try to obstruct my hearing somehow, using earplugs or headphones. If I can leave, I do leave. However, most of the time I'm triggered during class, so I can't leave. If I have to hear a trigger for too long, I get very overwhelmed and feel like crying. I've never actually cried, but I've come very close. Sometimes, to distract myself, I pinch my hand or arm. Never too hard, rarely ever hard enough to even leave a mark. It's always just hard enough to draw my attention to the physical sensation which can be very relieving compared to hearing a trigger.

Full of Sound and Fury

Interview 13: Cathy Bacchus

At what age did you start to have triggers for misophonia?

About 9 or 10.

What are your top 5 triggers?

Gum chewing (visual and sound), crunchy or mouth noises with food, tapping, bass or music or voice sounds (i.e., cars/neighbors).

What is worse, visual triggers or audial triggers?

Audial.

When did you learn that there was a name for your condition and other sufferers?

About 2006 or 2007.

How did it feel to learn that there were other people like you?

Didn't feel as crazy or alone.

How do you cope with this disorder?

Avoidance most of the time, stay inside my home, use headphones, noise machines, fans or earplugs.

Are your family and friends supportive?

When I was younger or before I knew – no.
Marriage break-up, etc. Some friends are supportive but do
not understand.

Are you afraid to confront a person when
they are triggering you?

Yes.

If a person does not respect your condition,
how do you react?

Anxiety, want to flee. If not, anger inside or self-
harm.

Do you have other disorders that worsen
your Misophonia?

Yes, anxiety, depression, OCD.

Do you think the name suits the disorder?

Why? Why not?

No, because I think it's more of a sensitivity-pain. It
gives me a physical reaction which causes fear, which is not
necessarily a hatred of sounds – it makes my body sick.

Explain the reaction when faced with a trigger:

I feel sick, my body twitches and I want to run away. I get tearful and feel like I am going to scream or explode in anger. I have caused self-harm to try and alleviate the strong feelings, or used drugs to get some sleep.

Full of Sound and Fury

Interview 14: Martin

At what age did you start to have triggers for misophonia?

8-9

What are your top 5 triggers?

- Chewing gum
- Chips cracking
- Popping gum
- Hearing my family members softly singing
- Hearing my neighbors' music

What is worse, visual triggers or audial triggers?

The same, but the audial are more frequent in my daily life.

When did you learn that there was a name for your condition and other sufferers?

About June or July of 2014 on a website called 9gag.com, in the comments section from a post.

How did it feel to learn that there were other people like you?

It was a weight off my shoulders. It almost felt like having a "superpower" and knew there were more people with it that can help you to control it.

How do you cope with this disorder?

I try to live day-by-day the most normally possible, always carrying my earbuds and, of course, I have to eat alone (at least when I'm with my family), because for some reason I don't get mad or annoyed when I hear my friends eat.

But most important, I think the music I listen to helps me a lot to calm or get rid of my rage. I listen to metal music.

Are your family and friends supportive?

Most of the time, they try to no eat anything when I'm near to them.

Are you afraid to confront a person when they are triggering you?

Not really. Usually, I'm a peaceful person and I would prefer to walk away.

If a person does not respect your condition, how do you react?

I don't really know, because only my family knows that I have it.

Do you have other disorders that worsen your misophonia?

No.

Do you think the name suits the disorder? Why? Why not?

No, because I think there is not enough medical studies to tell this must be a disorder.

What do you think could be done to raise awareness?

Make a viral campaign.

Explain the reaction when faced with a trigger:

First of all, when I notice the trigger, all my senses begin to sharp and unconsciously focus on the sound. Then I have to quickly see the environment I'm in; if I can walk away, I take that option, if not, I have to take out my earbuds and begin to listen to my music until I can get the trigger out of my head. If for any reason I don't have my earbuds, or just can't use them for being on my job or something serious, I turn my face into an angry glare and then I begin to stare the person who is making the trigger until they understand that I'm mad. If that doesn't work, I use my last resort ... begin to mimic the sounds or the trigger moves that the person is making.

And by the way, fortunately, I haven't reached the point that I want to punch someone for triggering me with misophonia-related things, in the worstcase scenario I just think that I would scream at the person to stop doing the trigger.

How To Cope

How do you cope with a disorder that most of the world, including doctors and researchers, don't know exists? In my experience, sufferers deal with this with great difficulty. I've heard of people trying radical methods to help cope with misophonia. Since it's so debilitating, many are willing to try absolutely anything to combat the negative aspects of the disorder. This chapter will discuss methods that have been used by people with misophonia, my own personal experience as well as any research or medical claims that back up a method, where available. Please understand that, while frustrating, there is currently no official cure for misophonia. These methods may help one person and not another. Your best defense against misophonia is to use trial and error and respect your journey to find peace of mind.

I used to think that avoidance was the best way to stay away from triggers. But I eventually realized that this was counterintuitive. When "missing out" on important events and socialization, I began to realize that this made me anxious and depressed. Then, I would be triggered more if I happened to be in the situation. Obviously, this isn't what we want to happen. Instead, it's important that we practice mindfulness and are aware of our limits but willing and ready to compromise, try and live a full life despite our limitations and our disorder.

Misophonia is not a life sentence

There's no question that misophonia changes the lives of those who suffer from it. It also changes the lives of parents, siblings, friends and romantic partners. This doesn't mean that you need to hide your entire life. Sure, it's hard to live with, but life is still possible with these complications. With a few adjustments, you can have a normal, fulfilling life.

You may have to change what your idea of "normal" is to match your needs. After all, life is about what you make it. Stop thinking of misophonia as something that has "happened to you" and start thinking about it as an interesting part of you. I know that can be hard to consider. After all, it sucks. But, think of it this way – this is a part of who you are, for better or worse.

Regulate, Reason, Reassure

Regulate, Reason, Reassure (RRR) by Dr. Jennifer Jo Brout is the most comprehensive (and only one I know of) coping skills program for misophonia to date. Using her own experiences with misophonia, her now adult child's experiences and years of clinical practice with misophonia patients, RRR is a truly fantastic manual that gives practical coping tips for misophonia.

Until there is a treatment – and perhaps even afterwards – RRR provides a reasonable framework for clinicians, adults and parents of children with misophonia.

On www.misophoniaeducation.com I assist Dr. Brout in running workshops, classes and educational events to help clinicians, parents and adults with misophonia learn coping skills as well as practical information on misophonia. These workshops provide insight on the disorder and are regularly co-hosted by guests such as Duke CMER's Dr. Zachary Rosenthal, amongst others.

RRR is far too expansive to explain in this brief section, however a summary could go like this:

Regulate: Get the sensory system back to baseline

Reason: Work through the emotions that come from the triggers (i.e., parsing out which sounds are reasonable/unreasonable, coming up with compromises, etc.)

Reassure: Finding reassurance such as in your own journaling, loved ones, clinicians or other ways that reinforce the view that the misophonic sufferer is more than their disorder.

The full coping skills manual is available on Amazon at the following link, https://amzn.to/3hVidwK and the description is below:

Regulate, Reason, Reassure: A Parent's Guide to Understanding and Managing Misophonia, is a coping skills manual for parents to help their own children and teens manage misophonia. RRR was developed by Dr. Jennifer Brout through her own experiences as a clinician, a sufferer of misophonia, and the mother of an adult child who showed signs of misophonia at a young age. RRR gives parents the tools to help mediate misophonia and provides easy to follow guidelines and work sheets to ensure parents have the skils to continue practicing RRR with their child as they grow and develop.

For those viewing the print version, it might be easier to simply search the title Regulate, Reason, Reassure: A Parent's Guide to Understanding and Managing Misophonia.

The Misophonia Provider Network

The Misophonia Provider network is run by the International Misophonia Research Network (IMRN) and Misophonia Education. The provider network is part of Dr. Brout and my efforts to increase understanding of misophonia. Providers listed must complete workshops from Misophonia Education and prove that they have at least the most basic level of understanding of the disorder to be listed.

General Coping Tips
Living a Healthy Lifestyle

No matter the disorder, I am a firm believer that a healthy lifestyle is our first line of defense. We would not want to send soldiers into battle malnourished, tired, sluggish and dehydrated. So, why then does it seem perfectly okay to stuff ourselves with cakes and soda and assume that our problems aren't becoming worse because of it? After all, our bodies are only able to work with the tools that they have.

I have been struggling with Anxiety and Depression for ten years. Through that journey I have learned that the most important tool for coping and our bodies is to understand that we are beings that live lives of connectivity.

I want to mention that the best help for misophonia right now is *Regulate, Reason, Reassure* and other coping skills. The following information is mostly my opinion and should be taken with a grain of salt. However, I don't think it is harmful or controversial to say "drink water, sleep and eat healthily" no matter the condition or lack of evidence on one condition in particular.

Water Intake

It isn't a coincidence that water holds a place at the top of this list. Water is absolutely crucial for a healthy lifestyle. I never knew how dehydrated I was for years until I started drinking an appropriate amount of water. Like a good shower, water has washed away a lot of the cloudiness from my life. Triggers aren't completely alleviated but I have more energy, am less stressed and I feel as though the world is a brighter place. There's never an excuse not to drink enough water, ever. I swear by the practice. In order to make it feasible, I use a free iPhone app called Waterlogged to track how much water I drink daily. I don't always meet my goal, and when I don't, I notice it quickly. The negative aftermath goes well into the next day. The rule I follow is to drink half your weight in ounces.

While some doctors and nutritionists have other ideas, this works for me. I feel so much better now that I drink a good amount of water every day. For example, since I am 150 lbs. right now, I drink at least 75 ounces of water a day. I usually exceed my goal by rounding up to 80 ounces. To make it easier, I measure my water in 20 oz. bottles and then pour it into a glass. Once I'm done with the entire bottle, I register it in the app.

Additionally, I measure my teacups. Each cup of tea is 10 ounces of water. I get a lot of my water from herbal tea which I used to hate. Remember, the feeling of thirst means you're already dehydrated. Drink water at regular intervals throughout the day. You may want to avoid drinking a lot before bedtime as a full bladder can lead to restlessness and an inability to sleep.

You may want more water depending on how you feel, or if you're very active. Listen to your body. If you're not sure about your daily intake, make sure you consult your doctor. Don't be afraid to ask questions that sound odd. It's perfectly reasonable to ask your doctor about your water intake. It's wise, even.

Diet

Misophonia may not be cured by eating right, but a lot of people who suffer from the disorder have noted that they feel much better, and are triggered less, when on a healthy and "clean" diet. On my fridge, I have a quote taped to the front. It reads, "You are what you eat. So, don't be cheap, easy and fake." High sugar and processed diets aren't doing you any favors. This is especially true if you are already dealing with a condition as strange and discouraging as misophonia. Perhaps eating right won't "cure" the illness, but eating improperly leads to stress on the body, and when you're stressed, you're more likely to be triggered.

Let's not forget the added risks of this highly processed diet: cancer, diabetes, hypertension, heart disease and many others. Beware—the modern diet hides sugar everywhere, and all of my research on health has led me to believe that all sugar is sugar, and sugar is bad. Some interesting books and documentaries highlight exactly why sugar is so deadly. Several doctors are now comparing sugar to poison and believe that sugar leads to a plethora of negatives.

In 1972, before much of the world had caught on, John Yudkin wrote a book explaining the dangers of sugar, entitled *Pure, White and Deadly*. Aside from being a university professor he was also had an M.D, PhD and M.A., Yudkin believed that, "The consumption of sugar on top of an ordinary diet increases the risk of obesity; the consumption of sugar instead of part of an adequate diet increases the risk of nutritional deficiencies" (55). If you want to avoid sugar you must be mindful, it is in nearly every processed food and "In the food industry, finding the bliss point for sugar in dinner products like pasta sauce would soon become passé. Products for meals were relatively easy" (Moss 103) and continue to be in these foods, and many more.

Personally, I feel much better now that I have incorporated a significant amount of vegetables, proper protein and reduced sugar, sodium and processed food intake considerably in my diet. It's important to believe that healthy food is not worse, or a punishment. When done right, healthy food is highly rewarding and delicious.

I would never recommend a fad or niche diet. I'm a firm believer in nutrition being a very personal thing. It is not a one size fits all ordeal. Some people are lactose intolerant, but others aren't. I eat milk, cheese and dairy, despite certain warnings. Personally, I have opted for organic options and I feel much better. But, it's up to you to determine your relationship with foods. You may want to practice mindfulness and explore what exactly is being pumped into your body at every turn.

Since there is little proof as to what exactly long-term chemical exposure, or even GMOs, are going to do to the body, I believe it is important to be considerate of these factors. That does not mean that you should make choices based on conspiracy theories but simply be aware. You should try different options and see what your body thinks about them. Let your mental and physical health be your guide for what is right for you.

As for cooking, it is an important part of the daily ritual. Much of modern life has become an avoidance of preparation and "busy work." But it is these exact activities that may help us to regulate our sensory systems. As well, preparing your meals yourself gives your body the proper chance it needs to prepare for food and aids digestion.

Exercise

The least fun out of any of these, exercise always seems to land at the bottom of every to-do list. Aside from some gym enthusiasts, exercise is seen as some form of modern torture. I have to admit, I'm not a fan. However, I won't dispute that for some, exercise can provide an amazing high. The endorphins released will help you to deal with stress, possibly triggers, and as a bonus, you'll be sweating out the toxins that can be harmful to your body. You don't have to train for a marathon or be an Olympic swim champion to reap the benefits of exercise. Start off slowly. Thirty minutes, three times a week of a physical activity that you enjoy will get the ball rolling, and the more you do, the more you'll feel able and willing to do it. Try to make exercise fun by bringing a friend along. A friend who understands your misophonia and who is willing to compromise will be best. You don't want to be trying to combat triggers while trying to de-stress. However, if you're already triggered, you can use exercise as a way to relieve the tension and beat out the anger. Think boxing.

If you push aside all your excuses, you're left with one fact: exercise will help to improve the overall quality of your life. When I first wrote this section, I was entirely unaware of the proposed benefits of sensory diets used by occupational therapists or the role exercise can play. Since learning this I have been considering all options and trying things that may help to regulate instead of just picking an exercise and going for it.

I like to choose things like swimming because I feel most comfortable in the water. But I live in Canada so this can be hard in the winter. That's when I enjoy things like bowling, skating or sledding. I'll admit it's hard to adjust to going out in public and being triggered at first, but, when you're bringing along friends and having fun, you may just forget that you're in a "high risk" environment.

Mental Health

So many of our emotions are tied to our state of mental health. A good mood can help you to push triggers aside. If you're happy, you're less likely to let a trigger bring you into a state of depression or heightened anxiety. Mental health can bring a trigger from feeling like the apocalypse to feeling like a bump on the knee. This is one way that a therapist can be beneficial. They may not understand misophonia, but they do understand how to help others to live a stress-free life and to make meaningful changes in order to feel happier and more fulfilled, despite any challenges. Co-morbid conditions like OCD, Anxiety,

Depression and ADHD should be treated by appropriate medical professionals.

The following are some ways in which your mental health can be helped:

Tips for Mental Health

Drink tea. Whether it's red, green or white, tea has been proven to have great benefits. It can significantly help to alleviate stress, and even help your digestion. This is also a great way to reach your daily intake of water. If you believe that caffeine has a negative impact on your misophonia, try herbal, caffeine-free teas.

Do yoga, or some other form of stress management. Yoga, Pilate, and other activities are great for your mind and your body.

Find things you love. When you're doing things you love, the bad doesn't seem as bad. Even if there are triggers momentarily, you are much more likely to recover in an environment that makes you happy.

Be creative. Creativity is like a cheap drug. You can paint, do crafts, photography, design and just about anything that lets your brain wander and find interesting ideas to incorporate into an artistic form.

Make goals and work toward them. When you're achieving life goals you will feel better about yourself. Especially when these goals are being met to spite your misophonia. It can be a small goal, such as a healthier lifestyle, seeing your mother more, or a goal as large as starting your own business. The point is that working toward your goal will be good for your mind and can help improve your life.

Use white noise. White noise is very important for eliminating audial triggers from an environment. Times like sleeping, being on a bus or simply in day-to-day life can benefit from the addition of white noise. White noise can be found in the form of noise apps for phones, videos on a computer, fans and white noise generators. Similarly, a TV or music may do the trick if you're merely trying to tune out trigger noises and cover them. There are also comforting sounds like ocean music and other "calming" sounds. White noise may be more effective because it tends to block out our ability to hear these noises altogether, but music or a TV show can be helpful by creating a positive mood. It really depends on what you're looking for. Regardless of the noise that you choose to go with, it is very useful to prevent hearing a trigger. White noise is most effective as a preventative measure but can help lessen the effects once already triggered. Avoiding trigger sounds altogether is the best outcome, but that's not always possible. Remember that white noise will not take away the anger and discomfort that you are feeling toward a trigger, but it will help you to not hear more of the sound.

Distraction

This can be highly beneficial when trapped with a trigger. When you're in a car, on a bus, in class or somewhere that you can't immediately leave, it's important to train your mind to focus on something else. It will not alleviate the entire trigger, but it can take your reaction from a ten to a two, if you're good at distracting yourself. You can distract yourself in many ways. Distraction is an important tool when you cannot get out of the situation. I have been known to put up my school bag as a barrier in class, in order to avoid movements, and I am also known for wearing earplugs in class or playing games on my computer or chatting up a friend on my computer when I am trying to get away from the trigger environment mentally. A friend can help via text or a chat service, and you can really alter your mindset by making the time go by faster. This will not completely alleviate the trigger, but it may make it a lot easier to deal with.

It's Okay to Grieve

Misophonia is a life-altering condition with no existing treatment aside from coping skills, therefore, it's important that sufferers focus on what this means for them. It is important not to push these feelings away and feel guilty for having them. Grief must be dealt with and allowed to go through its stages. Once you grieve, you can accept that this is not the end of the world and that you can still make a life for yourself. Grieving is not about giving up, it is about letting go, and moving forward with the changes that have to be made. There are five stages of grief that were originally proposed in the book *On Death and Dying* in 1969 by Elisabeth Kübler-Ross. The stages of grief do not necessarily happen in order, and you can go from depression back to anger or any other combination.

The 5 Stages of Grief

1. Denial and Isolation: Denial can come in different ways. People with misophonia may at first believe that they're just "hyper- sensitive" or that it's their fault.

Isolation is huge for misophonia. A large number of sufferers spend most of their time alone and choose jobs and activities where triggers will not bother them. While this may help to prevent triggers, it is not a meaningful way to spend all of your time. Personal relationships and social interactions are a large part of happiness. Alone time is great, but it should not be all of your time.

2. Anger: It makes sense to be angry with misophonia. It's a life-changing, existence-altering condition. Even when you finally find out that you're not crazy and there's a name for it, you're faced with a harsh reality. There's currently no cure, and that's enough to make anybody angry. Of course, it's not fair that you have to suffer from this and that you can't just be "normal." However, the fact is, you have it and you're going to have to move on. Yes, your anger is warranted. However, you can't risk the rest of your life and your happiness because of this condition.

3. Bargaining: Sufferers may try to find help in ways that have a small chance of working. This can involve using therapies that have either not been tested or approved or have little evidence to support that they will work. While these methods can be very helpful for personal acceptance, it is not helpful if done out of desperation. Lack of results may put you further down a path of anxiety and depression and heed your progress.

4. Depression: It's easy to get depressed when things seem so bleak. Misophoria has been known to cause depression so severe that hopelessness and thoughts of suicide are possible. If this happens to you, you should contact a mental health professional. It is important that you are properly equipped with coping mechanisms to help you through these emotions. Depression from grief is normal, but if it becomes too intense and endangers your life, medical attention is a necessity. Do not feel guilty or be afraid that you might be judged if you need to ask for help. It shows great strength to seek the help that you need. Whether through therapy or soul searching, you must process your negative emotions and come to terms with them.

5. Acceptance: After you have gone through all of the stages of grief, it is important that you come to a realization: There's nothing you can do to change things. It's all right. Misophonia may be a chronic condition but that does not mean that you will not be able to live a meaningful life. Once you accept misophonia, it will be easier to focus on coping methods and creating the kind of life that you want to live.

Misophonia-Friendly Activities

Living with misophonia doesn't have to be a trap. You can live a full and happy life while dealing with this disorder. The following are activities that can be enjoyed, especially in environments where triggers may be minimal.

Bowling: If you're okay with the sound of the balls rolling and the pins crashing, then bowling should be a good place to hang out with your friends. For those with visual triggers, it is usually dark during evening bowling nights, especially on "neon" or "blacklight" nights that often happen on weekends. A bonus is that music and the sound of the crashing will most likely block out any small trigger noises.

Swimming: It's exercise, and it's fun. Swimming can be a great activity for those with misophonia. However, you may not want to swim in a pool that is mostly filled with children if you do not like screaming. Also, some pools have lifeguards that are trigger-happy with their whistles. Find a pool or a public beach that has minimum or no triggers and you should be able to enjoy a meaningful experience with your friends.

Staying In: Staying in with your friends doesn't have to be a boring experience. You can play video games, play board games, watch movies, cook together, have a mini party and do whatever you enjoy at home, but with friends. This environment can be trigger-free if you pre-warn your friends and ask them to respect your boundaries.

Nature Hike: If you're in an unpopulated area you can enjoy nature with your friends and let the scenery sink in. A possible trigger may be the sound of the birds, but if that doesn't bother you, then you should be fine. Make sure that your companions are aware of your misophonia and are willing to abstain from behaviors that may bother you.

Malls: Hit-or-miss, depending on the nature of your triggers. But I love malls because I can easily get out of a situation if it triggers me. There are so many sections and stores that I'm never forced to be with the same people for very long. It's easy to go to another store and forget about what happened. However, some people find stores and malls very irritating.

Places With High Trigger Levels

Unfortunately, not all places are misophonia-friendly. These places will not trigger everyone but can be devastating for those that it does trigger. While now and then may be okay, some of these places should be avoided altogether if you are in a particularly heightened state beforehand. If things that go on in these places heavily trigger you, you should not try to force it. Sometimes we have no choice but to go to a place that will trigger us. Below each section there will be some tips for handling the situation if you find yourself forced to endure it, or if it is something you enjoy regardless of potential triggers.

You need to find your personal limits. Do not force yourself to stay home merely because there "may be" a trigger. After all, the world is an entirely huge place with lots of possibility. You may very well get hit by a car when crossing the street. Should you only ever go to stores on the right? Of course not. Risk is a part of life. Evaluate the risk of a situation based on your current mood and feelings. If you're having trouble seeing due to fogged glasses, you may not want to cross the road until a) you can get your glasses cleaned or b) another day when it is not foggy since you do not need what is on the other side very much. However, if you truly need something on the other side of the road, you may decide to "suck it up."

Misophonia requires checking in with yourself.

Theatres

Chewing, shuffling feet, people's silhouettes moving in the dark and maybe some seat-kicking. Depending on your triggers, the theatre can be a nightmare. However, some people find going to theatres can be manageable with headphones that are used for disabilities. You can contact your local theatre to ask if they offer them before going.

If you do go there:

- Try to use headphones for sound
- Sit near the back so that you do not have people behind you. Try to be near friends so you will not feel alone

Restaurants

Unfortunately, restaurants are breeding grounds for triggers. Both visual and audial triggers are in abundance at most restaurants. If you're lucky, you can find a nice booth in a quiet back corner, but if you're going during regular business hours, you may be in for an unpleasant experience. The only pleasant dining experiences I have had in restaurants in the past 2 years have been at odd hours, and when I happened to be the only patron. I recommend take-out, pick-up or delivery if you really want to splurge on restaurant food.

If you do go there:

- Try to sit away from the kitchen, there is a lot of noise from the workers
- Try to sit at the back of a booth with your friends on the outside to act as a buffer for triggers
- Get a table in a corner away from others
- Try to go at times when there are usually less diners, such as 3pm

Waiting Rooms

These places are full of triggers. People in waiting rooms tend to be anxious and their nervous ticks can become full-blown triggers for a person with misophonia. I try to avoid waiting rooms as much as possible. Waiting rooms are an unfortunate fact of life and should be avoided if they can. However, if you need to be in a waiting room, chances are you have to go there. If it is for a government document or paper, first check to see if you can get this service done via mail.

If you do go there:

- Sit in the back, or in a corner
- If you can, have a friend sit next to you in order to block out other people
- Try to book appointments in the early morning or mid-afternoon. These times people are usually at work and not at appointments

Public Transportation

Hot, stuffy and cramped with people. Public transportation, whether trains, busses or planes, is filled with misophonia triggers. Those of us who have no other choice are forced into this awful situation, sometimes multiple times a day.

If you do go there:

- Try to go when there are less people. If not possible, try to sit as far away from people as possible and isolate yourself. I usually put my backpack on my lap and look out the window

- Sit in the back, or in a corner
- If you can, have a friend sit next to you in order to block out other people

Be Wary of "Treatments"

Since there is no official treatment for misophonia, there may be people who claim that he or she can help sufferers to alleviate all of their symptoms. To a person who has been suffering all their life, these cures can sound like a miracle and mimic the trend of the dieting industry. These people are looking for your money, and they are not to be trusted. This does not mean that all "cures" are scams or fake, but it does mean that you have to be weary.

If a person approaches you offering a cure, you should not accept just because it seems like a miracle cure. Actually, you should be quite disgruntled as "miracle cures" do not exist for this condition. Most doctors do not approach patients; even researchers are unlikely to do so because they understand the ethics involved with offering experimental treatments. Unfortunately, a doctorate or medical practice does not mean that the person has significant working knowledge of misophonia.

Full of Sound and Fury

Explaining Misophonia

Since misophonia isn't a widely known disorder, it is important that those who suffer are well-equipped to explain their condition to parties who could be causing a trigger or to those who are able to provide support for misophonia. This chapter will aim to provide suggestions for explaining the condition to different parties and will suggest ways to avoid a negative situation. It is important that you feel respected by everyone that you interact with. Of course, this can be difficult when dealing with strangers – but when it comes to people you have a personal or professional relationship with, respect must be maintained.

Tip for all people you have to deal with: regardless of who it is, be assertive when you state that you have a neurological condition. You can be polite and assertive at the same time.

Explain that misophonia does not mean that you are making excuses for yourself, it merely means that you are taking your health into your own hands.

If a person does not understand but shows interest, offer to send them links to sites on misophonia. Tell them that it's reasonable that they don't know, but that there is growing research on the disorder. Before arranging to meet with a new person, I briefly explain my disorder. I explain that certain sights and sounds give me a fight or flight reaction and ask that they keep them to a minimum. I have had much more success explaining this before a meeting than in the moment when being triggered, which is essentially too late.

Friends

I now refuse to spend time recreationally with people who do not respect my misophonia. It was a hard adjustment at first – but the people who truly care about me are able to respect my condition. Friendship, like dating, should be based on a mutual understanding and trust. You should not have to pressure your friend to respect your needs and wishes, and your friend should not feel attacked by your sudden rage at noises or visuals. Be sure to explain to your friend that you do not mean anything by your displeasure, and that you truly value their time and your relationship. Ask if you can have gatherings in trigger-neutral zones and plan your outings so that the possibility of a trigger is minimal. This can be hard since a lot of friendships involve activities that involve noises or visual stimuli. Try to pick outings that have noises that you are comfortable with. For example, I'm fine with the sound of bowling balls and pins crashing. Bowling is a great way for me to hang out with friends because most of the people I can see are standing – which means not shaking any body parts, and the rest of the facility is usually dark. A great friend will understand that you are not doing this to be nitpicky and will want to make you feel at ease. However, you must understand that they have emotions too, and that you should try not to attack them when triggered.

Romantic Partners

Ah, romance, the place where we're supposed to accept the other individual regardless of their inconsistent behaviors. Misophonia is the devil in your ear nagging at you. Your partner clinks their spoon in a bowl, taps their fingers or shakes their leg. Maybe they like to whistle. At first, you may try to ignore it, but eventually the triggers can become worse and worse. The honeymoon phase is over, and misophonia changes all of your emotions. Like friends and family, you need to be able to discuss your misophonia with your partner. Hard work and honesty are going to be the key in going forward. Your partner must respect your condition and know the role it plays in your life, and you must understand and respect your partner's emotions when it comes to being the trigger and living their life with you.

Family

Those nearest and dearest are often the worst triggers. We spend a lot of time with our loved ones and, in general, we seem less forgiving when it comes to their behaviors. Day in and day out with the same people can be stressful for anyone. Even if you do not live with a family member, the intensity of the relationship can still cause misophonia triggers to be worse. My first ever "trigger person" that I knew was my mother. At first, every time she shook her foot it was a major fight. We're talking volcanic eruption on both sides. You didn't want to be there when she played music and when she sang. I know it isn't her fault that she does these things, and they never used to bother me. Misophonia doesn't always make sense.

Roommates

Like family, these people are there on a day-to-day basis. However, unlike family, there may not be enough of a personal relationship that you can confront the individual in a positive manner. Sometimes, our living arrangements are out of our control. You may be living in a dorm room, an apartment or another communal situation. Money and other uncontrollable forces often lead to the necessity of living with a stranger, or even an acquaintance. Ideally, we would never live with someone whom we didn't have a good relationship with. Unfortunately, reality isn't always a perfect picture. If you're going to be living with a new person, you should discuss your misophonia before moving in. Try to be sure that the person you're going to live with truly understands your needs and establish ground rules. Explain that you are not trying to dictate them and that you are merely suffering from a neurological condition. If they, or a current roommate, do not respect these ground rules, perhaps you should consider a different living arrangement if possible. Living with your triggers should only be a last resort. While you cannot avoid triggers in every aspect of your life, the home should be a neutral place where you can relax and have a sanctuary for the sake of your health and sanity.

Boss or Administration

Your boss should be a person that you trust and that you can approach with issues that involve your work performance and comfort in the workplace. For some people, their boss is intimidating and a person that they would rather not confront. Either way, it is best to go into this conversation prepared. You should explain misophonia is a neurological condition that can't be helped, though there is little information and no cure yet. Ask your boss if there is anything they can do to help, and assure them that you are committed to the job and are asking for the betterment of not just yourself, but your performance. If your boss is not supportive, you should be armed on the laws reflecting accessibility in your region.

Co-Workers

Co-workers can be tricky. You have to play nice when you have a job. This is especially worrisome for those that work in an office environment. A lot of workplaces are starting to allow snacking on the job, and this causes a lot of triggers. Being polite can go a long way with other workers, no matter the situation. However, sometimes coworkers aren't willing to stop something that they believe is "their right." Approach the co-worker when you aren't triggered and inform them that you have a medical condition and ask them if they would be willing to help accommodate you. If they are not willing to help and further the situation, inform your boss. You should already have told your boss about your misophonia and discussed the possibility of accommodations. If you are lucky, you may be able to convince your boss to speak with your co-worker. Remind everyone involved that misophonia a neurological condition that you cannot control.

Doctors (and other Medical Professionals)

When faced with a medical struggle, most of us decide to go to a doctor. The trouble with misophonia is that many doctors have never heard of it. Most doctors will automatically assume that it is psychological and will refer you to a psychiatrist or a psychologist, or personally recommend medication. This can be frustrating and possibly infuriating. Depending on where you live, it may cost a lot of money to be thrown through hoops without knowing if you'll ever find a cure. It's best to do your research on doctors that provide help for misophonia. However, you should still have a conversation with your doctor and let them know what is happening with you. As research grows, your doctor may become interested in the illness and could eventually help others, and maybe even you.

Teachers and Professors

For those of you lucky enough to be out of the school game, I salute you. Dealing with professors and teachers can be its own kind of hell. Thankfully, most schools these days (at least Universities, Colleges, and Technical Schools) have great accessibility programs. They're not perfect, but they're getting a lot better. The hardest part of this seems to be intimidation. The entire system seems set up to make professors and teachers seem larger than life, and that can be intimidating. If your school wants you to discuss your condition with your professor, you must approach them when you are in a good mood. You should never approach your professor on a day on which you are triggered. I have been lucky enough to only have positive interactions with my professors in regard to my misophonia, anxiety and depression. Remember that most teachers and professors are there to help you. They are not the enemy and they want their students to succeed. All of your interactions should be polite, considerate and professional. Speak to the professor with kindness but firmness.

Going Into the Conversation

When you know that you have to tell a person about your disorder, it can be stressful – the anxiety, fear and anticipation can be enough to keep your mouth firmly shut and continue your suffering. However, it's important that you go through with it. Keeping things bottled up will not help your disorder or your life – I promise you that. Consider the tips below when you're going to confront somebody. You may want to adjust the conversation depending on whom you're talking to, but these tips should help you when thinking about how to act, what to do and what to say. It's a good idea to make sure you're not triggered at the time of the conversation. During a trigger, your anger is heightened and you may perceive the person as a threat. It's important that you are prepared to explain misophonia in a positive manner. No one wants to feel attacked.

Prepare yourself with research and website links that can be help to explain misophonia to the person you're about to approach. Make sure that they will understand that it is a real condition, and that you are serious.

Keep your mood stress-free and ensure that you are relaxed beforehand. Try to have a bath, some tea and some light television or something you enjoy before you have the conversation. If you're stressed or tired, the conversation may go south quickly. It is important that you are in a good mood for the conversation. Choose a location in which you know there will be little to no triggers. Try to be somewhere that you and the other individual are both comfortable. If this is not possible, try to become familiar with the place beforehand (such as talking to the person in their office and asking if you can meet another day, when you have more time or are more prepared).

During The Conversation

During the conversation, your aim should be to keep it positive and informative. You should provide examples of what trigger you, even if they are not the *same ones* that trigger you in the environment with the person. It's important that they understand it is not just when you are around this person and that this disorder impacts several aspects of your life. Do not make it all about them.

It may be helpful to print off articles that explain misophonia and what it is. Despite research being minimal, some of the websites listed at the end of this book can be helpful for learning about misophonia. If the person triggers you during the conversation, identify it but not in an aggressive manner. Excuse yourself and explain that what they are doing is one of the things that cause a reaction. Politely ask if they can stop or if there is a way they can adjust their behavior. Make sure they understand you are not blaming them, but that the condition is serious.

Do not apologize for misophonia or make excuses. Say that it is a neurological condition and that you have it. Be matter-of-fact and explain that, unfortunately, there is no cure.

Discuss a way that you can let them know you are being triggered without being offensive or turning to anger.

If the conversation starts to go sour or the person does not understand – excuse yourself. Do not let anger turn into a confrontation. Explain that you were merely explaining your feelings and that this has a huge impact on your life. Leave before it becomes more serious, often leaving is a statement of its own.

After the Conversation

Chances are, after you explain misophonia to another person they will still trigger you. It can be hard for a person to recondition things that they are used to doing, and even harder to remember. Unlike you, this person does not deal with misophonia on a day-in-day-out basis, so it's unlikely that it's something they consider regularly. Do not blame them for this and do not hold it against them. Unless the person is trying to trigger you and disregards your feelings entirely, you should be mindful that they are probably not out to get you, and that is merely a reaction from misophonia.

- If you have to remind them that they are triggering you, be polite

- Leave the room and if they ask why, explain that you're being triggered
- Try to remain positive; do not engage when you are angry

The Other Side of The Fence

I get it, explaining misophonia to another person is a hard thing to do. It can send us into a panic. We don't want to be judged and we're worried about the reaction of the person we're confronting. But, have you considered what the reaction of the other person may be, and why? I know you're worried that there will be a lack of understanding and a negative reaction – but why would it be negative?

Hearing a sufferer explain her condition and also how she changes her lifestyle for her son gave me some ideas. For once, I wasn't the person explaining that I had the disorder; I was merely the person listening to the story. As well, I've read all the interviews in this book and had conversations with a lot of sufferers. To say the least, it was strange to be on the other side of the fence. This is the side where you don't exactly know what to say, and you're at a loss for words. In this section, I want to shed some light on this position. Hopefully, I can also help people without the disorder to understand what they could say to get around their confusion. There's a good chance that the person who is triggering you does not want you to feel such a negative reaction from their behavior. Even worse, they may feel guilty or like they're being blamed for your thoughts and feelings and that can be troublesome to live with. The following are considerations to make about the feelings of people who are your triggers, and what it may be like to be them.

I haven't always had misophonia. I can still remember the days of old when I wasn't bothered by or triggered by any noises. A person who doesn't have sensory processing issues or misophonia probably won't notice the sights or sounds that you're noticing. In fact, they may be so oblivious that they don't even know if they're making noise or moving. When you have misophonia it's nearly impossible to imagine that these noises or visuals can be completely unseen and unheard. However, when you're not living with it on a daily basis, it can be very hard to understand what the big deal is about. A person without misophonia may wonder why you're so upset and first think you're merely hypersensitive. It's not their fault that they think this way. Each person has trouble seeing outside of his or her own experiences, so it's hard to consider the viewpoint of a person with misophonia.

A person who is triggering a loved one or a close friend may feel a significant amount of guilt when trying to deal with misophonia and its impact on their loved one. After all, they do not want to hurt you. And yet, one wrong move and they're being given the stink-eye, again. It's traumatic to always be griped at and "attacked" for making a noise you're used to or moving a part of your body. Unfortunately, the person who is triggered has little control of their rage in the moment. However, that doesn't mean that the feelings of the person who the rage is directed toward do not feel it too. People have trouble considering changing their habits or behaviors in order to ease the lifestyle of another. It's not because they're arrogant or selfish, it's because everybody is just trying to get by in their own way. A significant amount of the population hums, whistles or shakes their legs or sways when they are uncomfortable or faced with anxiety. Unfortunately, these behaviors tend to send people with misophonia into a rage, and this reaction could further send the person causing the trigger into anxiety. Misophonia is uncomfortable for everybody involved.

The lack of medical knowledge and research on misophonia is not only challenging, but also very confusing for people who do not have it. If you think it's hard living with the disorder, imagine watching it happen but not knowing what to do, or whether or not your actions could actually be making the disorder worse. This is especially challenging for parents that are trying to guide their children in the right direction. A lot of people will say that their kids cannot be coddled and that they should be forcing them to "toughen up." This can send a mixed message to parents. Since the pain associated with misophonia is severe, a parent's reaction will be to protect their child – but a lot of people will be urging them to force their child to "get over it." All current findings on misophonia indicate that the disorder gets worse with exposure. It'll be impossible to keep a child away from any and all triggers but forcing them to deal with it is not the way to go. There's a fine line between avoiding life and purposefully exposing a person to triggers. Balance should be sought that helps each person, and there is no "one-size-fits-all" approach to take care of misophonia.

Misophonia is an emotional struggle for everybody involved. There are no right answers, and the current amount of research and diagnosis is so small that it's hard to feel a sense of hope once you know that it's, in fact, a real diagnosis. However, this does not mean that everything has to be gray skies. Open communication can be helpful for everybody. If you are being triggered, you should be able to communicate this positively or, if that is the only excuse available, leave the room. If you are not the person suffering, but rather the trigger, or a person involved with a misophonia sufferer, you should learn not to take their behavior personally.

Here are some things to think about, in regard to misophonia. This is broken into two sections. The first is for loved ones and the second is for sufferers. I recommend you each read both so that you can get a full picture of the situation. Understanding is an important part of having a harmonious relationship.

For Loved Ones

If you are triggering your loved one, do not treat them as though it is simply his or her problem and that they have to get over it. Acknowledge that it is a real problem and, if you are unable to adjust what you are doing, at least be mindful of their emotions.

If your loved one leaves the room or excuses his or herself from an event or a conversation, either momentarily or for long periods of time, try not to make them feel guilty. Misophonia is very sensitive to exposure and it should be encouraged that the person feels safe and comfortable in finding the right balance for his or her life. It is important that a person with misophonia knows that they are able to escape and that they are not trapped or isolated in the situation.

Try not to feel guilty. It is not your fault that your loved one has this disorder. However, even if it is your actions causing the trigger, it is not your fault that this is happening, it is misophonia that causes this reaction, and you have nothing to feel guilty for.

If you are experiencing difficulties explaining misophonia to other family members or friends who do not understand the reaction of your loved one, explain to them that it is a neurological condition and that your loved one's brain simply interprets certain noises and sounds differently than others, and that they see them as a threat. Explain that this reaction is usually both physical as well as emotional, that the rage is felt immediately and that they are unable to control it.

Consider family counseling. Although a counselor will not be able to cure misophonia, they may be able to help your family develop ways of understanding each other. Misophonia tends to lead to a self-centered attitude in sufferers due to the nature of the disorder. It can be helpful to have a therapist that understands at least some sensory processing issues. It is important that you and your entire family know how to communicate and express emotions in a positive and mindful manner.

If it's been a heated day for you and the sufferer, consider taking a mini-vacation from them. This may involve watching a movie in another room or removing you or the sufferer from the environment. While you're apart, it can be nice if you're both doing something you love and enjoy. When you come back together, you may both be ready to talk in a calmer manner or, at least, without taking each other's throats out.

For Sufferers

You must remember that your loved one has emotions too. Yes, you are angry and triggered by an action. However, your loved one is impacted by this disorder as well. Significant life changes happen on both sides and it is important that you are mindful of their sacrifices and the negativity that they must deal with. Even though it is not your fault that you feel this way, you cannot discount the other person's feelings.

You shouldn't feel guilty for leaving a family event or a friend's house. If you have to get out of a situation, that's that. Unlike anxiety, it will not help you to push through a trigger. However, if a trigger is not going to last long, like fireworks, a brief scene on TV or other momentary things, it is reasonable to stay. However, if you are being consistently triggered and feel your mood getting worse and worse and your angry heightening, it may be wise to get to safer pastures and wait out the storm.

If your misophonia is causing a rift in a relationship, try not to feel guilty. While you cannot change how you act in a trigger situation, or at least not a lot, you can change how you behave after the situation. Be mindful of the emotions of the other person and be sure that you're willing to negotiate parameters and ground rules for how you deal with the situation. Having a plan can help everybody involved know what's going to go down, and there will be fewer hard feelings afterwards. Any bumps that do happen can be discussed instead of fought over.

As mentioned in the section above, family counseling can be a great way to help everybody talk through their feelings and discuss their emotions in a positive and effective manner. If therapy is not available because of cost or other restraints, you can simply Google ways to discuss important family matters or come up with a plan that works best for your family, then sit down and talk it out.

Another repeat from the "Loved ones" section: take a break from the person who is triggering you. Go to a friend's, go to your own room or go for a walk outside. It's not helping anybody if you're staying in a negative situation.

Awareness

Since misophonia is only a newly recognized condition, it is important that the doctors who study it, and the people who suffer from it, are advocating for awareness. Some believe that awareness will lead to negative individuals acting inappropriately against sufferers, but with proper advocacy, this should be alleviated.

Awareness is important for all disorders and conditions. This is evident in the growing support for mental illness and the need for open dialogue and understanding. Of course, it is not possible for the entire world to change in order to help those who have misophonia, but through awareness we will further incentives for research and for plans that can genuinely help those with misophonia.

In my own experience, misophonia has been much easier to manage now that I can tell family and friends what is wrong. Like a good diet, healthy and understanding friends and family can lead to an overall improvement in quality of life. It's important that the people you interact with know that there is currently no cure. Therapy might help, but it will not eliminate symptoms.

Once upon a time, many of the disorders we are now aware of and actively working to alleviate today were considered abnormal and strange. Misophonia may currently be considered abnormal or strange, but as awareness grows, this may become a stigma of the past. There may be an initial period of downfall. The more awareness grows, the more it may be considered odd and a piece of gossip. All things must go through this phase. In order to have gains we must be prepared for the potential losses.

Awareness isn't some magical concept that can be achieved simply by wanting it to happen. If we want misophonia to be a widely understood and accepted condition, we must be willing to talk about it. Like all illnesses that have been stigmatized, it starts with a conversation.

It can be difficult to talk about misophonia. There's a lot of pressure when you know that the person on the receiving end probably won't understand what you're going through. That doesn't mean you shouldn't try. Everyone can help raise awareness for misophonia. It starts with your family and friends, your community, your school or workplace. At first, it may be seen as a strange word, a strange disorder or an annoyance. Over time, it will grow to be something familiar. Information and exposure are the only way that a person's mind can be changed. Of course, there'll always be the naysayers, the doubters and the people who refuse to respect your illness – but these people exist in all lifestyles, for all reasons. There was once a time when it was okay to label a disabled person as retarded. Now, that's so unspeakable that I considered using asterisks for some of the letters. There was also a time when people with depression and anxiety were told to suck it up, and there was a time just few decades ago where these people may have spent their lives in an asylum. The world is changing, but it isn't changing through suffering in silence.

It is my belief that access to information is an important way to spread word about this illness. Posts that can be shared, posts featuring information and graphic images, can help those who suffer from misophonia to share information with their friends and families. For me, what's most important is that people know that this is more than a condition and a label; misophonia is a life-altering disorder that can seriously impede a person's quality of life. This book was written for the purpose of awareness. It is through information that we will change how the world views this disorder.

In *Beyond The Label*, stigma is discussed in detail. Stigma is more than just how a person feels about a disorder, it has a great impact on the life of the sufferer. While misophonia is not the same as mental illness, there is little else to compare it to – and since the reactions appear mental (to an onlooker), it can be put under the same umbrella as many mental illnesses. Below is the definition of stigma in a book designated to raising awareness and cutting away the label for mental illness and addiction.

Stigma is not merely a problem of "hurting people's feelings." Stigma interferes with the person's full participation in society, can lead to and/or increase mental health and substance use problems and can provoke the person to withdraw from relationships and services that could be helpful. Stigma can seriously hamper matters such as holding a job, having a home, accessing services and participating in social relationships (CAMH).

The fear of being judged and scrutinized can stop people from looking for help. Since misophonia is not a well-known condition, attempting to search for a cure can be very isolating, which may be worsened when sufferers find out there is none. This is why awareness is so important – awareness can remove stigma, both from the medical community and from the public. Without research, misophonia will remain a relatively unknown condition, and without advocacy, demand will remain low. The more doctors, graduate students and people have heard of misophonia, the greater the chance of finding meaningful treatment or helping sufferers to handle the disorder properly.

Here are some ways that you can help raise awareness for misophonia.

Social Media

You may think that social media's best attributes are sharing game invites with friends and connecting with your long-lost childhood friend. That may be true, but it also offers a plethora of resources for raising awareness. The ability to post, like and share has allowed many organizations to get their messages across. The more that people hear about misophonia, the greater the chance that doctors and researchers will learn about it.

Social media is an amazingly powerful platform. Anybody, anywhere, at any time, can connect and share a vision and an idea. It is easy to spread awareness and content with people whom you may never have met without social media. Through Twitter, Google + and Facebook you can reach a wider audience and ensure that the message of misophonia gets out there. I recommend that you follow the Misophonia International/Misophonia Education page on these sites and share our content with your friends and families.

Your Community

You may be surprised to learn that your own community holds opportunities to raise awareness. You can ask to set up an information booth at functions, whether these are BBQs, advocacy events or merely community parties. You can raise a lot of awareness by having pamphlets, posters and other items ready to promote awareness.

Friends and Family

Your friends and family can constitute a great backdrop for explaining your disorder. Remember that each person you inform will be able to tell another, and then another. Simply explaining misophonia to others can be both cathartic and a way to spread awareness.

Your School/Workplace

Like the sources mentioned above, you may be surprised about the awareness you can spread just by talking to your workmates/classmates, and other professionals. These people may also have great resources that you can take advantage of. This provides a wonderful opportunity for networking. Besides, you never know what somebody will be working on down the road, and how you can be mutually beneficial to one another.

They are:

Respect the person as an individual. Chances are they are not trying to trigger you, and merely have little to no understanding of the disorder.

Try not to approach a person who is triggering you with a discussion on misophonia when you are triggered. If you must say something, take a breath and remain calm. Politely ask the person to stop. Do not verbally attack the person.

Understand why the person makes the noise and do not disregard their feelings. Say you understand, but that it is a medical condition and that you would really appreciate if they would be willing to help you.

Do not apologize for your disorder. This takes away credibility and makes it seem like there is something you can do differently.

My Advocacy Journey

There is an awkwardness in writing about your work and your professional life. Despite that awkwardness, I am making an attempt to put into words what feels like four decades, despite only spanning from 2015 to 2021. It is especially weird to talk about my advocacy journal in this book because the first edition of *Full of Sound and Fury* marked the beginning of my advocacy journey with misophonia.

I felt compelled to write this book, and share the stories of fellow sufferers, because at the time there was very little information about misophonia, and a great deal of confusion and self-loathing was associated with the disorder for many that had it. Luckily, there is a lot more research and hope today than there was when I first wrote the book in 2015. I am forever grateful to the researchers who are committed to exploring misophonia and finding answers in these uncharted waters.

Misophonia Awareness

Misophonia Awareness was a website that provided information on how to advocate for misophonia as well as basic information on the disorder. This website has been discontinued as Misophonia International and other projects grew and took its place. While awareness is still important, it has taken a backseat to research and education as academic and clinical information on misophonia has grown.

Misophonia International

Misophonia International started as an ambitious project. Dr. Jennifer Jo Brout and I decided to start a news site and print magazine for misophonia. I'm still a little shocked by our commitment to this leviathan of a project. Though I was a web and print designer at the time, I had never done anything on this scale, and there was a lot of learning on the spot—and a lot of late nights freaking out.

Since the original launch, Misophonia International has changed to be a coping, news and awareness site exclusively. We share articles from sufferers, doctors and researchers. The print magazine portion of the site—which was a little *too ambitious*—has been discontinued with articles archived in the anthology *Exploring Misophonia* which is available on misophoniaeducation.com or on Amazon in print or eBook format.

Misophoniainternational.com continues to be a project dedicated to providing updates on misophonia and also provides product reviews (such as headphones, weighted blankets, sensory toys, etc.) by sufferers.

Writing and Articles

From a young age I have considered myself a writer. I've always loved putting things into words, and many of my goals were oriented around publishing books. This book was my first, and I am grateful that it helped me on the path I had always envisioned for myself. Lemons and lemonade, if you know what I mean. However, this wasn't the only adventure in writing I have taken—I have spent a great deal of time dedicating my efforts to writing about misophonia.

On July 26th, 2016 my first "official" article was published on another platform. I published *When Sound Is Sinister: I Have Misophonia* in The Huffington Post. This was the first of many publications on misophonia including articles for Huffpost, Thought Catalog, Different Brains, The Mighty, and Physician's Weekly, amongst others.

I am grateful for these opportunities to share my thoughts and help advocate for misophonia to a wider base.

How We Survive Ourselves

As a writer, I have always had an affinity for fiction. While advocacy is rewarding, I love telling stories and making up worlds. *How We Survive Ourselves* is a combination of advocacy and fiction. You can find a preview for this novel at the end of this edition.

How We Survive Ourselves tells the stories of mental illness through the eyes of a man with dissociative identity disorder, a young woman with misophonia, a young woman with depression, the wife of the DID sufferer and a therapist trying to help these characters cope. *How We Survive Ourselves* is meant to be a realistic picture of mental illness, but that does not mean there is no hope. Through the eyes of the characters and their experiences, a new sort of understanding develops.

My first fiction novel, *Acceleration*, was not an advocacy endeavor, so I was really excited to write a book about misophonia, DID and depression. Although, I must say I was also nervous to write a book with advocacy in mind. That said, I am so happy that I wrote *How We Survive Ourselves* and I can't wait to write more books that will hopefully help people understand disorders.

Misophonia Providers

Misophoniaproviders.com is a provider network that lists providers for misophonia around the world. Providers must complete education from misophoniaeducat.com to be eligible to be listed. The goal is to help persons with misophonia find clinicians who have at least a basic understanding of misophonia. This site is run by the IMRN, Dr. Jennifer Jo Brout, and technologically run by myself, Shaylynn Hayes.

Misophonia Education

Our latest project is misophoniaeducation.com which provides classes (Regulate Reason Reassure), workshops and informative events led by doctors and researchers. The majority of workshops are presented by Dr. Brout, and we have recurring events from Duke's Center for Misophonia and Emotion Regulation (CMER).

This project feels like a cumulation of all our work and I am so happy that we can finally provide education and coping skills to clinicians, parents of misophonia children and misophonia sufferers.

I personally run the technical side of Misophonia Education and provide tech support, design and produce the workshops. In the future I hope to expand my reach and finish a counselling degree so that I, too, can help educate.

Conclusion

Strangely, I did not feel compelled to write a conclusion for the first edition of this book. I suppose I was young and edgy and saw no need for the formality of a conclusion. Regardless, I now feel compelled to write a concluding chapter and summarize my thoughts and feelings on misophonia as best as I can.

My message of conclusion is very simple: there is hope in misophonia research, in coping skills and in the increasing education and information that has been championed since 2015. I am especially grateful for the misophonia work of Dr. Suhkbinder Kumar, Mercede Erfanian, Zach Rosenthal, Clair Robbins, Lisalynn Kelly and many others who have joined in the cause of misophonia advocacy and research.

Education, research and coping skills are the key to living a functional and fulfilling life with misophonia—and I hope this updated version provided some much-needed hope.

Shaylynn Hayes-Raymond

References

Ahn, R., Miller, L. J., Milberger, S., &McIntosh, D. N.
(2004). Prevalence of parents' perceptions of
sensory processing disorders among kindergarten
children. American Journal of Occupational
Therapy, 58 (3), 287-302.

Alvarado, J.C, Vaughan, J.W, Stanford, T.R., and Stein,
B.E. (2007). Multisensory Versus Unisensory
Integration: Contrasting Modes in the Superior
Colliculus. Journal of Neurophysiology 97, 3193–
3205.

Ben-Sasson, A., Carter, A.S., & Briggs Gowan, M.J.
(2009). Sensory over- responsivity in elementary
school: prevalence and social-emotional correlates.
Journal of Abnormal Child Psychology, 37, 705-
716.

Ben-Sasson, A., Carter, A.S., & Briggs-Gowan, M.J.
(2010). The development of sensory over-
responsivity from infancy to elementary school.
Journal of Abnormal Child Psychology, 38 (8),
1193-1202.

Carter, A.S., Ben-Sasson, A., & Briggs-Gowan, M.J.
(2011). Sensory over- responsivity,
psychopathology, and family impairment in school-
aged children. Journal of the American Academy of
Child & Adolescent Psychiatry, 50 (12), 1210-1219.

Davies, P.L., Chang, W-P., & Gavin, W.J. (2009).
Maturation of Sensory Gating Performance in
Children with and without Sensory Processing
Disorders. International Journal of
Psychophysiology, 72, 187-197.

Davies P.L., Chang, W.P., & Gavin, W.J. (2010). Middle
and late latency ERP components discriminate
between adults, typical children, and children with
sensory processing disorders. Frontiers in
Integrative Neuroscience, 4, 16.

Davies, P.L. & Gavin, W.J. (2007). Validating the
diagnosis of Sensory Processing Disorders using
EEG technology. American Journal of Occupational
Therapy, 61 (2), 176-189.

Edelstein, M., Brang, D., Rouw, R., Ramachandran, V.S.
(2013). Misophonia: physiological investigations
and case descriptions. Frontiers in Human

Neuroscience 2013;7(296), 1-11, doi: 10.3389/fnhum.2013.00296.

Gavin, W. J., Dotseth, A., Roush, K. K., Smith, C. A., Spain, H. D., & Davies, P. L. (2011). Electroencephalography in children with and without sensory processing disorders during auditory perception. American Journal of Occupational Therapy, 65, 370–377.

Goldsmith, H.H., Van Hulle, C.A., Arneson, C.L., Schreiber, J.E., & Gernsbacher, M.A. (2006). A population-based twin study of parentally reported tactile and auditory defensiveness in young children. Journal of Abnormal Child Psychology, 34 (3), 393-407.

Jastreboff, M.M., Jastreboff, P.J. (2001) Hyperacusis. Audiology Online. www.audiologyonline.com/articles/hyperacusis-1223.

Jastreboff, P.J., Jastreboff, M.M. (2006) Tinnitus retraining therapy: a different view on tinnitus. International Journal of Pediatric Otorhinolaryngology, 68 (1), 23–29.

Keuler, M.M., Schmidt, N.L., Van Hulle, C.A., Lemery-Chalfant, K., & Goldsmith, H.H. (2011). Sensory overresponsivity prenatal risk factors and temperamental contributions. Journal of Development & Behavioral Pediatrics, 32 (7), 533-541.

Kisley, M.A., Noecker, L., Guinther, P.M. (2004). Comparison of sensory gating to mismatch negativity and self-reported perceptual phenomena in healthy adults. International Journal of Psychophysiology, 41, 604–612. doi: 10.1111/j.1469-8986.2004.00191.x.

Lane, S.J., Reynolds, S., & Thacker, L. (2010). Sensory over-responsivity and ADHD: differentiating using electrodermal responses, cortisol, and anxiety. Frontiers in Integrative Neuroscience, 4 (8), 1-14. doi:10.3389/ fnin.2010.00008.

McIntosh, D.N., Miller, L.J., Shyu, V., Hagerman. (1999). Sensory-modulation disruption, electrodermal responses, and functional behaviors. Developmental Medicine & Child Neurology, 41, 608-615.

Owen, J.P., Marco E.J., Desai S., Fourie E., Harris J., Hill S.S., Arnett A.B., Mukherjee P., (2103) Abnormal white matter microstructure in children with sensory processing disorders. NeuroImage: Clinical, 2, 844–853.

Rosenthal, M.Z., Ahn, R. & Geiger, P.J. (2011). Reactivity to Sensations in Borderline Personality Disorder: A Preliminary Study. Journal of Personality Disorders, (25), 5, 715-721.

Schaaf, R.C., Miller, L.J., Seawell, D., & O'Keefe, S. (2003). Children with disturbances in sensory processing: A pilot study examining the role of the parasympathetic nervous system. American Journal of Occupational Therapy, 57.

Schneider, M.L., Moore, C.F., Larson, J.A., Barr, C.S., DeJesus, O.T., & Roberts, A.D. (2009). Timing of moderate level of prenatal alcohol exposure influences gene expression of sensory processing behavior in rhesus monkeys. Frontiers in Integrative Neuroscience, 3, 30.

Schröder, A., Vulink, N., Denys, D. (2013) Misophonia: diagnostic criteria for a new psychiatric disorder.

PLoS One, 8 (1). doi: 10.1371/journal.pone.
0054706.

Tavassoli, T., Miller, L.J., Schoen, S.A.Nielsen, D.M.
&Baron-Cohen S. (2014). Sensory over-
responsivity in adults with autism spectrum
conditions. Autism, 18 (4), 28-32.

Van Hulle, C.A., Schmidt, N.L., & Goldsmith, H.H.
(2012). Is sensory over- responsivity distinguishable
from childhood behavior problems? A phenotypic
and genetic analysis. Journal of Child Psychology
and Psychiatry, 53 (1), 64-72.

Wu, M.S., Lewin A.B , Murphy, T.K., Storch, E.A. (2014)
Misophonia: incidence, phenomenology, and
clinical correlates in an undergraduate student
sample. Journal of Clinical Psychology. Published
online April 17. doi: 10.1002/jclp.22098

www.ingramcontent.com/pod-product-compliance
Lightning Source LLC
Chambersburg PA
CBHW070113030426
42335CB00016B/2135